Understanding Cancer

Understanding
Cancer

A Patient's Guide to Diagnosis,
Prognosis, and Treatment

SECOND EDITION

C. Norman Coleman, M.D.

Forewords by Edward C. Halperin, M.D.,
Vice Dean of the School of Medicine,
Duke University Medical Center, and
Ellen L. Stovall, Executive Director,
National Coalition for Cancer Survivorship

The Johns Hopkins University Press
Baltimore

Note to the reader: This book is not meant to substitute for medical care of people with cancer, and treatment should not be based solely on its contents. Instead, treatment must be developed in a dialogue between the individual and his or her physician. This book has been written to help with that dialogue.

The author and publisher have made reasonable efforts to determine that the selection and dosage of drugs discussed in this text conform to the practices of the general medical community. The medications described do not necessarily have specific approval by the U.S. Food and Drug Administration for use in the diseases and dosages for which they are recommended. In view of ongoing research, changes in governmental regulations, and the constant flow of information relating to drug therapy and drug reactions, the reader is urged to check the package insert of each drug for any change in indications and dosage and for warnings and precautions. This is particularly important when the recommended agent is a new and/or infrequently used drug.

© 1998, 2006 The Johns Hopkins University Press
All rights reserved. Published 2006
Printed in the United States of America on acid-free paper
9 8 7 6 5 4 3 2 1

The Johns Hopkins University Press
2715 North Charles Street
Baltimore, Maryland 21218-4363
www.press.jhu.edu

Library of Congress Cataloging-in-Publication Data
Coleman, C. Norman.
Understanding cancer : a patient's guide to diagnosis, prognosis, and treatment / C. Norman Coleman. — 2nd ed.
    p. cm.
Includes bibliographical references and index.
ISBN 0-8018-8417-9 (hardcover : alk. paper) —
ISBN 0-8018-8418-7 (paperback : alk. paper)
1. Cancer — Popular works. I. Title.
RC263.C64 2006
616.99'4 — dc22   2005033961

A catalog record for this book is available from the British Library.

Illustrations by Jacqueline Schaffer.

To my parents, Samuel and Minna Coleman;
to my wife, Karolynn, and my children, Gabrielle and Keith;
and to my patients, who have taught me a great deal
about what really matters in life.

Contents

Foreword

Edward C. Halperin, M.D.
Vice Dean of the School of Medicine
Duke University Medical Center

Why have you picked up this book? It's probably because you or someone you care about has recently been told they have cancer. How do I know this? Let me tell you a story.

I write and edit two medical textbooks. One of these books focuses on the treatment of cancer in children. When the book's first edition was published, I did what any faithful child and sibling would do: I sent copies to my parents and my sisters. One of my sisters leafed through the book and then left it lying on the coffee table in her living room. A few weeks later one of her friends was visiting her house. While they were chatting, the friend inquired, "Is everything alright?"

My sister responded, "Of course."

"How about your children? Are they fine?" the friend persisted.

"Yes, they're fine," my sister answered. "Why are you asking me these questions?"

"I can't stand it anymore," the friend blurted out. "I saw that book on your coffee table. Nobody would have a book like that lying around the house for leisure reading. There must be something terribly wrong. You must tell me."

"Calm yourself," my sister reassured her friend. "My brother wrote the book. He sent me a copy."

I relate this story because it is instructive regarding human nature. Cancer is a common public health problem. One would hope that interested citizens, being moderately scientifically literate, would read books about cancer, cardiac disease, diabetes, and other public health issues to be fully versed in the problems facing modern society. Unfortunately, almost none of us do it. We only turn our attention to matters such as cancer when they directly affect us or a member of our family. It is for this reason that I think it fair to conclude you are paging through Dr. Coleman's book because of an immediate and deeply felt concern over your own well-being or that of someone you care about. If my presumption is correct, then I am sorry you face this problem, but I think I have a few words that can help.

When confronted with cancer, most of us launch into an information-seeking behavior pattern. We begin, of course, by asking probing questions of our own doctor. Those of us with ready access to the Internet will begin scouring the Web, where we will encounter some reliable sources of information and much consummate nonsense. We next turn to printed health education brochures, the advice of friends and acquaintances, and our own intuition.

Health education psychologists teach us that many of us have difficulty with the assessment of risk. Most of us glaze over when faced with statements such as, "There is a 28 percent chance of relapse without chemotherapy and a 24 percent chance of relapse with chemotherapy. The chemotherapy has a 3 percent risk of mild to serious side effects, and we are not sure whether the chemotherapy affects the overall survival rate." The analysis of statistical measures of risk over time is a formidable challenge.

Faced with our fear engendered by cancer and our desire to be knowledgeable health care consumers, we need reliable places to turn. Although your first line of defense will be your own personal health care team, I am pleased to tell you that you can, with confidence, also use the book you are now holding in your hands. This is the second edition of *Understanding Cancer*, by C. Norman Coleman. I have employed the first edition for many years as a required textbook for Duke University School of Medicine students taking a fourth-year medical school course in oncology. Dr. Coleman provides his readers with clear explanations, appropriate examples, and concrete and usable advice, and he packages it all in an easy-to-read, easy-to-hold, and easy-to-understand book. He cannot tell you what is the best therapy for you. What he can and does do, however, is provide you with a framework for coming to grips with the diagnosis of cancer, knowing what questions to ask, and coming to a decision about what course of treatment, if any, you feel comfortable with.

The word *doctor* derives from the Latin verb *docere*, meaning "to teach." Dr. Coleman has fulfilled the role of teacher admirably, offering wise counsel and clear prose. The Hebrew word for doctor, *rofe*, means "to heal," in the sense of repairing, the mending of a tear, or the sewing of a garment's seam. It requires actively *doing something*—taking charge of the situation. As you read this book, you will be taking an active step toward healing by becoming knowledgeable at the feet of a wise teacher.

I am sorry that you or someone you care deeply about must now face the diagnosis of cancer. We may all take comfort, however, in the fact that every day, in clinics and laboratories throughout the world, an army of devoted physicians, laboratory scientists, health prevention experts, nutritionists, and epidemiologists are devoting their time and energy to the prevention, diagnosis, and treatment of cancer. We will eventually overcome this plague. Today, many are cured and others will have an extended, good-quality life. In the future, our children and grandchildren will endure less suffering and have less to fear from cancer than our generation does. For the present, I wish you strength in dealing with the diagnosis of cancer. This book is a good way to begin the process of understanding and healing.

Foreword to the First Edition

Ellen L. Stovall
Executive Director
National Coalition for Cancer Survivorship

I met Norm Coleman in the summer of 1993 when I was appointed as the consumer member of a federal panel mandated to evaluate the National Cancer Program and issue a report to Congress. I grew to have enormous respect and admiration for all fifteen members of that eclectic panel—a former congressman, a pharmaceutical company executive, several multidisciplined scientists, and cancer care specialists. But Norm Coleman was the one member of that panel who made me feel as though he had learned something from me—a twenty-six-year cancer survivor.

Since then, Dr. Coleman and I have continued to share our experiences as doctor and patient in an increasingly complex and rapidly evolving cancer research and health care marketplace. Through those conversations, I have come to know him as someone who knows how to listen, to learn, and to seek solutions that empower others to find answers that best address their needs in the face of a cancer diagnosis.

Many similar "how to" guides have preceded this one. But few have offered the distilled clarity that Norm Coleman offers cancer patients here. In these pages they will find relief in his realistic and understandable explanation about the goals of cancer treatment. He guides the reader through the quagmire of cancer treatment decision making by making the patient a part of the process. This may seem simple to someone who has not had to endure this exhausting exercise. It is far from simple, and one of Dr. Coleman's outstanding talents is his ability to simplify complex information. This arms the reader with vital information and renders the medical system, which is not always as user-friendly as we would wish, far less intimidating.

As a two-time cancer survivor (Hodgkin's disease diagnosed in 1971 and a recurrence in 1984), I am all too familiar with the rough terrain we patients must cross when making crucial decisions that will affect both the length and the quality of our lives. Cancer changes everything. It can turn our lives upside down and render us temporarily immobilized by the sheer weight of the diagnosis. Every day in my professional role, I meet men and women who feel paralyzed by the myriad treatment options confronting them. Now, at last, they have an invaluable map of that daunting terrain here in Norm Coleman's book.

A physician I know who read the first draft of this book admitted how little he had understood about how to explain survival statistics. As a result, he had been reluctant to discuss them with patients for fear of misleading them. When pressed, he would resort to saying "It's either 100 percent or nothing when it's you"— a response that satisfied neither his patients nor himself. He realized how much he could learn from this book. I hope many of his colleagues will follow his lead and turn to this book often.

Understanding Cancer: A Patient's Guide to Diagnosis, Prognosis, and Treatment will stand as a prominent asset in the vast bibliography of books on cancer. Norm Coleman shares with us his ability to verbalize, humanize, analyze, and, to the degree possible, normalize the entire cancer experience for patients, their physicians, and the team of family, friends, and caregivers who play supporting roles in the lives of those of us with cancer.

This book is written by a physician who has devoted his life to curing the ills of ignorance about cancer. That is his gift to us, the readers. As readers, our gift is to share it with others who will learn what Norm Coleman has taught us—that cancer is a lesser foe in the light of knowledge. With that knowledge comes understanding; with understanding, fear diminishes; in the absence of fear, hope emerges; and in the presence of hope, anything is possible.

Preface

Much has changed in clinical oncology since the first edition of this book was published 8 years ago. The era of molecular medicine was just beginning, with the improved understanding of the specific defects that transform a normal cell into a cancer cell. Today, drugs that target these defects, called molecular-targeted therapy, are commonly seen in clinical trials; one, Gleevac®, demonstrates the efficacy of this general approach in a disease called chronic myelogenous leukemia. Many more molecular-targeted therapies are in use and on the horizon. Cancer remains a complex disease in which there are multiple abnormalities in the cancer cell, however, and the cell can undergo further mutations that may make ineffective a drug that had been effective. So, the cat and mouse chase continues.

Combinations of treatments and new approaches—including the use of drugs and radiation together, immunotherapy, less invasive surgical techniques, improved imaging modalities, the simultaneous use of multiple drugs, and the application of new technologies to ablate the tumor—make the multidisciplinary approach to research and treatment ever more important. Molecular biology techniques are so far advanced that we can use the molecular signature or profile of an individual tumor to help select treatment. We have entered the era of personalized medicine.

All of these exciting advances have been accompanied by the rising cost of health care, which is a serious issue for all of us. To help determine the appropriate use of new therapies, there is an increase in the application of practice guidelines based on evidence-based medicine. The availability of many new treatments provides a much greater number of options for each patient, but it also exposes the patient to the pressure of sorting out what is a proven advance versus what is an exciting press release. The Internet is now a common source of information that can barrage us with facts, advertisements, hype, and hope—all mixed together. Thus, people with cancer and their families have an even greater need to be able to *understand* medical concepts, doctor-speak, scientific jargon, and analytical concepts. Access to new treatments requires patients to give more serious consideration to participating in a clinical trial, and clinical trials are now done in a much more complex regulatory environment than they were a decade ago.

All of these developments explain why the Johns Hopkins University Press and I decided that this is the time for this new edition of *Understanding Cancer,* and I am most appreciative of their interest in making the information in this book available to you—people with cancer and their family members. This book is meant to help you become an educated consumer in a short period during a tense time in your life.

I have used this book as part of a successful seminar series for basic scientists called TASC (Take a Scientist to the Clinic), at the National Cancer Institute. This seminar includes two or three one-hour discussion seminars and a half-day spent with a clinician during a patient evaluation. The term *translational science* is used to describe science that goes from the bench (laboratory) to the bedside (patient) and back, with the emphasis on clinical application (treatments). This book helps provide translational scientists with a "patient's-eye view" and has assisted other medical professionals who are interested in oncology decision making to better understand what a patient goes through and to improve how they communicate complex information to patients.

This second edition of *Understanding Cancer* includes all of the information in the first edition, with significant updating for the new era of molecular and personalized medicine. A new chapter on molecular-targeted therapy has been added. Feedback from readers remains important and is encouraged. In the last 6 years, I have returned to the National Cancer Institute (NCI) as director of the Radiation Oncology Sciences Program after 14 years at Harvard Medical School. I continue to see patients and I maintain a laboratory research program. Working in the NCI also offers a broad view into the future of cancer care and the issues facing cancer research; in this book I share my view with you. The preparation of this book is independent of my work at the NCI and should not be interpreted as indicating policy or opinion of the NCI or National Institutes of Health (NIH).

Understanding Cancer

Introduction

Dealing with the complex health care establishment and medical procedures can be very difficult, even when the medical problem is a minor one. And the need to understand unfamiliar medical terms and scientific concepts increases the burden. For people who have cancer, the situation is even more difficult and confusing, because anxiety makes it harder to digest all the information that comes their way. Even when there is an excellent chance of cure, the life of a person with cancer becomes extremely complicated in a hurry.

It is very hard for people who have just been told they have cancer to concentrate on much of anything at first. If you are like many people, not only are you trying to cope with the detailed information your doctors are giving you but you are also feeling bombarded by conflicting information from the Internet, newspapers and magazines, and radio and television. It can also be confusing and distressing to hear stories from family members and friends about what happened to people *they* know.

During many years of working with people with cancer and their families, I have found that one of their greatest needs is to understand the medical terms used in cancer care and the scientific concepts behind cancer and its treatment. Understanding terms and concepts is even more important in the era of molecular medicine, managed care, and rapid advances in diagnosis and treatment. That is why I wrote this book: to help people with cancer understand what they hear, what they read, and what they experience. This book describes the steps that people with any type of cancer are likely to go through during their diagnosis and treatment. In the process, it explains the terms and concepts used by health care professionals.

For the person with cancer, the information in this book will help prepare you for visits to doctors and the hospital and will make those visits more productive. When a choice of treatments is available, I hope this book will help you gather and interpret information about the different treatments, help you have more productive discussions with your doctor, and help with decision making.

I encourage patients to learn as much as they can about their illness and treatment, but some people don't want to know the details. Their attitude is, "You're the expert, Doc. I'll do whatever you say." Although this feeling is understandable, it is not generally helpful. The amount of information that each person wants to know is different, but knowing at least some basic facts and concepts about the disease and the treatment will help you as well as the person providing you with medical care. To handle the medical aspects of cancer as well as possible, you need to become knowledgeable about the disease and its treatment. That's why another goal I have in writing this book is to allow patients to explore information about cancer at their own pace, so they can avoid two unpleasant situations: information overload and the feeling that they have lost control of their situation.

Most people, understandably, know more about how to make a decision about buying a new car or a home appliance than about how to make decisions about medical treatment. We all know that a person doesn't need to be a mechanic to understand the basics of how a car or an appliance works. Similarly, one doesn't need to be a doctor to deal intelligently with cancer and its treatment. People with cancer are faced with decisions and different alternatives far more often than they realize at first. By acquiring a modest amount of knowledge, you and your family will be able to participate more actively in decisions about your medical care and will find that the time spent with your doctors is more valuable.

Most doctors try to provide complete information to their patients, and most patients and families try to listen carefully and ask sensible, necessary questions. However, lack of time makes it impossible for any doctor or any other health care professional to provide all the detailed information a patient and family really need to make informed decisions about treatment. While this book can't provide specific recommendations about your particular medical problem and its treatment, I hope the information in this book can help you work with your doctor and other members of the health care team to plan a course of care that will be best for you. The book will give you the tools you need to understand your illness, and it will serve as a guide to help you understand what you are likely to be doing at different times and in different settings. You will also find other excellent sources of information referred to at various points throughout the book.

A final purpose of this book is to serve as a *reminder* of what your doctor and others have already discussed with you and as *preparation* for what will happen next. It will make suggestions about what questions you may want to ask during your next visit to the doctor or the hospital.

One very important point: Because researchers have not uncovered all the facts about cancer, your doctors may not be able to answer all your questions. This is frustrating, and it can be upsetting. But it may help to know that some questions *can't* be answered, as much as your doctor wishes that he or she had all the answers for you.

Help for Nonmedical Aspects of Cancer

When people receive a diagnosis of cancer, they face the prospect of their own mortality. In addition to experiencing a natural fear regarding their own future, they are concerned about matters such as how their children will be cared for, how the disease will affect their careers, how it will affect other family members, and how the financial stresses that are often associated with cancer will be handled. Help with these nonmedical difficulties is available from doctors, nurses, social workers, psychologists, members of the clergy, and other members of the health care team. In addition, a variety of support groups and advocacy groups are available for people with cancer and their families. One excellent source of information is the National Coalition for Cancer Survivorship, at 1010 Wayne Avenue, fifth floor, Silver Spring, Maryland 20910 (see Chapter 1 for additional sources of information and support).

Addressing the nonmedical difficulties associated with the illness of cancer is an integral part of cancer care. Over the course of diagnosis and treatment, sometimes the medical issues will be most important, and other times the nonmedical issues will come to the foreground and will be most in need of your attention. This is a natural rhythm, and to be expected. And, just as medical issues have to be dealt with, so do nonmedical ones. I urge all people with cancer to seek and accept assistance from professionals who have experience helping with practical and emotional issues.

Cancer Survivorship

Currently, more than half of all people with cancer are cured of their disease, and many more live *with* cancer for years and years. With so many long-term survivors, a whole new set of psychological and social issues and concerns has come to the fore. Understandably, many survivors experience anxiety after they have successfully completed treatment. For one thing, survivors are afraid that the cancer will recur. They also experience a sense of loss, because they no longer receive all the support that doctors and other members of the health care team provided during the period of their diagnosis and treatment.

Some survivors discover that the stresses associated with the cancer diagnosis and treatment have strained their relationships with the people who are closest to them. Serious illnesses do put a strain on relationships, and yet the effect of some stresses can be minimized. There are professionals who can help with making the personal and family adjustments that cancer requires, beginning soon after diagnosis. Help is available at most cancer treatment centers from various members of the health care team and from support groups for patients and their families.

Many cancer patients, health care workers, and policy makers have only recently become aware of a variety of other issues that cancer survivors face, such as employment discrimination and difficulty obtaining or retaining health or life insurance coverage. As these issues gain attention as part of the national debate on health care reform, many cancer survivors, through local and regional organizations, are trying to remedy social and financial inequities and to increase governmental support for cancer research. The National Coalition for Cancer Survivorship (NCCS) is one of these groups. Many patient advocacy groups have already had a positive impact on prevention, screening, and treatment programs and have helped to educate the public and health care professions about the important issues facing cancer survivors. The National Cancer Institute's Office of Cancer Survivorship (http:// dccps.nci.nih.gov/ocs/) has information available and sponsors research on cancer survivorship issues.

A Word on Alternative, Complementary, and Unconventional Therapies

In this book I will focus exclusively on the cancer therapies whose effectiveness has been proven through scientific experimentation and research. But many nonstandard cancer therapies — ranging from vitamin treatments, special diets, and herbal medicines to relaxation techniques, bioelectromagnetics, and massage — are receiving increased attention from the medical community. Nonstandard therapies — also sometimes called *alternative, complementary, unconventional, unproven, unorthodox,* and even *unsound* or *questionable* therapies — interest people with cancer for a variety of reasons. Here are some guidelines I think are useful when thinking about these therapies.

People may hear about unconventional therapies from their physician or from sources outside the standard medical system, particularly the Internet. A physician, for example, may suggest that, in addition to undergoing conventional therapy, a patient might find relaxation therapy or meditation helpful to overall well-being; the physician will probably provide the name of individuals who can teach these techniques to the patient. Visualization techniques are useful for many patients in controlling chronic pain and getting through uncomfortable medical procedures, and many doctors encourage their patients to use these techniques. Some doctors can teach these techniques to patients; others provide a referral to someone who can. Even something as simple as listening to an audiotape through earphones can provide a welcome distraction. A physician may suggest a specific change in diet to help prevent the side effects of a treatment such as radiation. An improvement in general health that comes from eating a healthy diet and exercising can be very important for people undergoing cancer treatments (the person to consult about diet is your doctor or a professional nutritionist).

When the suggestion for an unconventional therapy comes from someone other than a physician, however, and whenever you are seriously tempted to undergo an unconventional or unorthodox treatment, my strong advice is to discuss the matter first with your doctors. Doing so may prevent a potentially dangerous interaction between the unconventional treatment and your standard treatment. The risks and benefits of the unconventional treatment must also be considered carefully, just as you will carefully consider any standard treatment before deciding to go ahead with it.

The answer to the question "What do I have to lose?" can be surprising. People who choose to rely on an unconventional therapy face a number of risks: (1) some of these therapies are dangerous; (2) a person may miss out on the benefits provided by standard treatment if he or she uses an alternative treatment in place of standard therapy; (3) questionable therapies almost always involve substantial out-of-pocket payment of cash that could be used to better advantage elsewhere; and (4) the person may lose precious time that could be spent on more worthwhile activities.

Another possibility with very serious potential consequences is that the patient, rather than the therapy, may be blamed if the alternative therapy fails. Some of my patients who relied on questionable therapies that failed were told that the treatment was unsuccessful because they did not follow the treatment regimen properly. As a result, these patients not only were faced with a serious medical condition but also felt a deep sense of guilt because they were unable to control their cancer.

Because almost all treatments that might help patients have been subjected to an objective review by the medical community, it is highly unlikely that someone would be *cured* by an unproven therapy. Some unproven therapies are helpful in providing relaxation or relief of symptoms; some do no harm but also do no good; and some unproven therapies harm people in various ways. There is an important medical concept called *evidence-based medicine* which applies to all aspects of medical intervention. Evidence-based medicine is used to establish practice guidelines, such as those of the National Comprehensive Cancer Network (NCCN). This concept means that there should be solid evidence that a procedure, medicine, or other therapy actually does what it is said to do. Such evidence comes from careful clinical investigation and assessment. For oncology, evidence-based medicine is relevant to both conventional and unconventional interventions and supports the need for clinical trials (discussed in Chapter 8).

Detailed information about complementary and unproven therapies is available from the American Cancer Society and the Office of Cancer Complementary and Alternative Medicine (OCCAM) at the National Cancer Institute. The best course is to develop an open and honest relationship with your doctor, so if you begin to feel frustrated or in other ways become unhappy about your situation, you and your doctor can work together to improve your care.

How This Book Is Organized

Different people have different needs for information at different times. The chapter titles and the major headings within each chapter will help you decide which chapters or sections within chapters you will want to read immediately and which ones you may, or may not, want to read later.

— A number of steps are involved in the diagnosis and treatment of cancer. These steps are reviewed in Chapter 1. Because these steps, or variations of them, apply to all patients, I urge all readers to read this chapter carefully. Most of the remaining chapters expand on the information in this chapter.

— Cancer is an extremely complex disease. Understanding this complex disease involves understanding how a normal cell behaves and how a normal cell becomes a cancer cell. Chapter 2 explains these processes and also examines the issue of whether cancer can be inherited—a concern that many people have. Appendix A provides additional details on cancer molecular biology.

— People with cancer must undergo a variety of laboratory tests and diagnostic imaging studies such as x-rays and other, more sophisticated imaging techniques. Chapter 3 explains why these tests are so important.

— Chapters 4 and 5 explain how the outcomes of treatment are measured and how to weigh the benefits of treatment against the risk of treatment, or the risk of having no treatment. You will need this information to make your own best possible decisions about treatment. As you will discover, doctors can only estimate the outcome of treatment; they can't predict the future for any individual. The information in these chapters is somewhat complex, but it is impossible to overstate its importance. It will help you and your doctors choose the treatment that is most appropriate for you.

— Three standard (conventional) treatments are currently available for people with cancer: surgery, chemotherapy, and radiation therapy. Most people are reasonably familiar with these treatments. In addition, several less common treatments, such as bone marrow transplantation and immunotherapy, are available. Each of these treatments is discussed in some detail in Chapter 6.

— Chapter 7 provides new information on molecular-targeted cancer therapy. This information is based on the background on cancer biology presented in Chapter 2 and in Appendix A. Molecular-targeted therapy and personalized medicine will change the face of cancer care in the coming years.

— Some patients benefit from participating in clinical research trials designed to test new treatments or modified versions of standard treatments. Chapter 8 describes the care with which these research studies are designed, the protections provided for participants, and the pros and cons about participating in such trials.

— Chapter 9 presents four patient stories, to demonstrate how a person can collect information needed to make an informed and appropriate decision about the treatment or treatments. These patients have different cancers, different life circumstances, and different treatment options. Their stories—their clinical cases—illustrate a range of possibilities for people with cancer.

— For readers who want more information, Appendix A explains cancer molecular biology in some detail, and Appendix B describes how cost-effectiveness is analyzed. Appendix C includes two commonly used systems for describing a patient's ability to perform the tasks of daily living. A checklist for patients is included in Appendix D.

— The bibliography lists some materials readers can turn to for more information on a number of issues.

I wrote this guide for you and your family, so that you can be active partners with your health care providers. I welcome any comments that might improve or enhance it. In the afterword you'll find information about how to contact me with your suggestions.

Chapter 1

Diagnosis and Treatment:
What You Can Expect

Τ his chapter provides an overview of the general processes involved in the diagnosis and treatment of cancer. It will describe the medical steps you are likely to go through, as well as some of the things you and your family will experience personally because of the disease. The "bird's-eye view" presented in this chapter will help you know what to expect and will allow you to plan ahead as much as possible. Most of the topics in this chapter are described in more detail later in this book.

Whenever anyone develops an illness that is going to involve tests, procedures, and treatments, it's very important for that person to gather all the vital information together in one place, so there is a reliable record that can be consulted along the way. The Patient's Checklist on pages 18 and 19 will give you an idea of the kind of information you will want to record and retain for future reference. Appendix D provides a copy of the checklist with plenty of space for you to organize and keep track of the details of your own diagnosis and treatment. There is space on the checklist for you to write down the information you gather as you progress through diagnosis and treatment. The checklist can be photocopied, or you can write directly in this book.

The steps that you will be likely to take during diagnosis and treatment are illustrated in figure 1.1, which also indicates the type of information you will need at different steps. You will almost certainly work on more than one step at a time, as you and your doctors gather information and decide which course of treatment is most appropriate. For example, you may make new arrangements for after-school child care while you are scheduling diagnostic studies. Or, while staging studies are under way, you may be seeking information about the health care professionals you'll want to consult once the results are known. There will be new terms to learn and new information to work with.

As you learn more about your cancer, you'll probably discover that there is more than one reasonable treatment option available to you; this is true of most cancers. The four patient stories in Chapter 9 demonstrate how different people make different decisions for different reasons and in different ways. As these cases help illustrate, there is no one decision that is perfect for everyone, and yet at some point you and your doctors will need to reach a decision and move on to treatment.

During the first few weeks after the diagnosis is made, there is much to do while you prepare to decide on a treatment and begin treatment. This preparation involves personal as well as medical matters. Because few cancers need to be treated as emergencies, you will have time to obtain the information you need and to prepare yourself for treatment. Although the various steps described in figure 1.1 concerning "medical" matters and "personal" matters are described separately, many of them can be attended to at the same time. We'll begin with the medical matters.

Medical Steps in Diagnosis and Treatment
Obtain a Diagnosis

Whether your cancer is diagnosed during a routine medical examination or during a visit to your doctor because of symptoms you're having, your family doctor or internist will probably be responsible for determining your diagnosis, often with the help of a surgeon, who may perform a biopsy by removing a small piece of the tumor. A pathologist will then examine the characteristics of the tissue under a high-powered microscope.

The diagnosis consists of naming the cancer, identifying where it began, and determining whether other parts of the body are affected. (Chapter 3 describes how different cancers are named and how their organ of origin is identified.) For example, a cancer of the breast is called an *adenocarcinoma of the breast* because of the

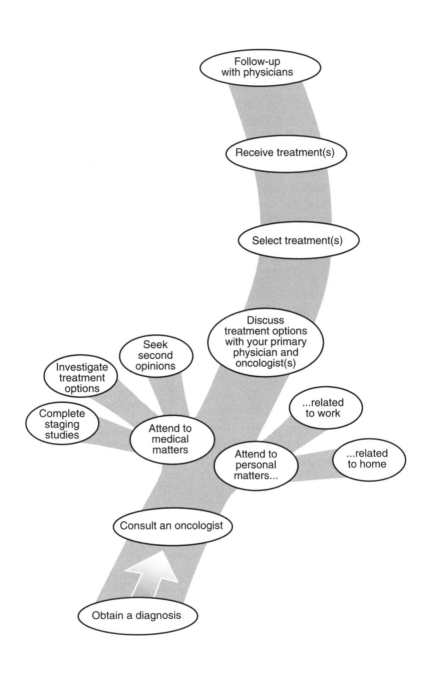

type of cell affected (glandular cell). A cancer that begins in the breast is called *breast cancer* no matter where it is found—that is, breast cancer that has spread, or *metastasized,* to another part of the body is still called breast cancer, because it began in the breast.

Consult an Oncologist

Because there are many types of cancer and many complicated treatments, your family doctor or internist probably does not have all the specialized knowledge needed to treat your illness. However, your family doctor *will* be able to help you arrange a consultation with an oncologist—a physician who specializes in the treatment of cancer. Your family doctor may or may not transfer the primary responsibility for your care to the oncologist, but in either case he or she will probably remain involved and may help you select your treatment. The doctor who has primary responsibility for a specific patient's care is called the *primary doctor.*

As you know, cancer is a complex disease. Because of this, more than one oncologist will probably be involved in your treatment. There are many different kinds of oncologists, and all of them have specialized knowledge about the diseases they treat. Their titles reflect their specialties, either the type of treatment they use or the type of cancer they treat—or even the type of patient they

---

Fig. 1.1. Steps in diagnosis and treatment (opposite)

After you have obtained a diagnosis and consulted an oncologist, the next steps involve both medical and personal matters. The medical steps will likely require a number of visits to undergo additional diagnostic studies and to see other physicians. The information you will gather will come primarily from the medical experts but also from other sources. The medical steps will likely take a few weeks or more, and you may find that time is well spent dealing with personal matters relating to home and work. As the medical and personal issues are being worked out, it is valuable to remain in touch with your primary doctor and primary oncologist(s), who will help you and your family reach a treatment decision. The close working relationship with your health care providers will be important to help you through treatment and will be a source of support and guidance when treatment is concluded and the follow-up period arrives.

treat. *Surgical oncologists,* as one would expect, specialize in surgery. *Medical oncologists* specialize in *systemic* treatments such as chemotherapy or immunotherapy, which involve drugs that are circulated by the bloodstream to attack the tumor. *Radiation oncologists* treat the tumor with radiation, and *pediatric oncologists* specialize in treating children with cancer. Some oncologists specialize in cancer affecting a specific organ, such as the breast or the lung, or a specific system, such as the lymphatic system. A doctor who specializes in cancer of the urological system would be called a *urological oncologist.* One who specializes in disorders of the blood is a *hematologist.*

As noted above, your primary doctor may be either your family doctor or an oncologist. You will also have a *primary oncologist,* who may or may not be your primary doctor. Your primary oncologist will help decide which treatment is best for you and will coordinate your care with other doctors.

Complete the Necessary Staging Studies

Your doctors need the information provided by staging studies to determine which treatments are best for you. Establishing the *stage* of the tumor (see Chapter 3) also provides a description that makes it easier for doctors to communicate with one another to coordinate your care.

The staging studies are performed to determine these things about your disease:

1. the site of the cancer
2. the size of the tumor
3. other parts of the body that may be affected by cancer cells
4. the treatments that are likely to be appropriate
5. the prognosis — how the disease is likely to respond to treatment

The prognosis is only an estimate of how a specific individual will respond to treatment. (This is discussed in more detail in Chapters 4 and 5.)

The two types of staging studies, clinical and pathological, are discussed in Chapter 3. Suffice it to say here that *clinical staging studies* include blood tests and diagnostic imaging tests such as x-rays, nuclear medicine scans, ultrasonography, computerized tomography (CT) scans, and magnetic resonance imaging (MRI) studies. *Pathological staging studies* are performed when it is necessary to obtain additional biopsies of tissues such as lymph nodes or bone marrow, or of tissue near the tumor.

An important part of selecting a treatment plan is to consider the natural history of a specific cancer—how the cancer is likely to behave if it is not treated. Is it likely to spread? If so, what organs are likely to be involved? How long will it be before symptoms develop? Because treatment is selected on the basis of how a particular cancer behaves, doctors need to understand its pattern of behavior—and that's part of the information that staging studies supply.

Most people are surprised when they learn that some cancers grow so slowly that immediate treatment is not necessary. For example, certain cancers involving the blood or lymph system which develop in older people don't cause problems for many years, even without treatment. Because no treatment is justified unless it is likely to result in a better outcome than would be the case if the disease were left untreated, people with such cancers have a good reason to defer having treatment. They may do extremely well without immediate treatment, though they must be watched closely by their doctor and receive treatment if a problem develops.

Seek Second Opinions

While the necessary staging studies are being performed, you are likely to see several different oncologists. Your family doctor may refer you to a large cancer center where you can get several expert opinions, for example, or you may go to such a center to receive treatments that require the expertise of several different specialists.

Once your situation has been assessed by one doctor, any plans or opinions obtained from other doctors are usually referred to as *second opinions*. A second opinion may agree with the first opinion, but, like many other medical experts, cancer experts do not always agree on what treatment is best for a specific patient, and it's likely that the second opinion will be somewhat (or even very) different from the first.

An important fact to keep in mind during this extremely difficult period in your life is that more than one treatment is reasonable and acceptable for some cancers. That's one reason why it is often a good idea to consult several specialists before deciding which treatment will be best for you and your situation. You absolutely have the right to do that, although you may find it difficult to do it if you are enrolled in some health plans. Doctors are used to having people seek second opinions, too, so you needn't worry about hurting their feelings or otherwise upsetting them. In rare instances, there may be very little time for second opinions. Otherwise you should feel free to seek another opinion if you choose to do so. It is not appropriate for you to be made to feel guilty about such a request.

There are two types of second opinions. In one, the second doctor you consult may have the same expertise as the first one. For example, if you see a surgical oncologist first, you can consult another surgeon to satisfy yourself that the first surgeon's recommendations are reasonable. In the other kind of second opinion, the second doctor you consult may have another specialty. For example, after seeing a surgeon, you may want to consult a medical oncologist or a radiation oncologist.

Second opinions are especially important when more than one type of treatment is available: for instance, if you are weighing surgery versus radiation therapy or chemotherapy versus radiation therapy. In addition, for many cancers, the appropriate treatment requires more than one specialist. Because cancer and its treatments are so complex, you need to understand the pros and cons of the different treatment options available to you. Your primary oncologist can be of great help to you while you are making a decision about treatment.

Gather Information about Treatment Options

Because few cancers require immediate treatment, you should have plenty of time to gather the information you will need about treatment options before you actually begin treatment. Even if the disease initially represents a medical emergency, a temporary measure will be taken to relieve the crisis and allow time to prepare for the longer course of treatment. Obviously, any prolonged delay in starting treatment is unwise. However, no one should make a snap decision about treatment because of self-induced panic or pressure from doctors or family members to make a choice.

The information you will need about each treatment option available to you includes answers to the following questions. You will obtain this information during your discussions with your doctor or doctors:

— How often will the treatment be given? For example, how many cycles of chemotherapy will I need?

— Where will the treatment be given? For example, will I need to be hospitalized?

— How will the treatment affect my job? For example, will I have to take time off from work?

— Will I be able to meet my family responsibilities? For example, will I be able to carry my infant?

— What side effects (complications) of the treatment can I expect? For example, will the chemotherapeutic drugs make me nauseous?

— What are the expected benefits of the treatment? For example, what are the chances that my disease will recur?

The Patient's Checklist will be extremely helpful in collecting information about and recording the answers to these questions. In addition to including the name of your cancer and the results of your staging tests, it will contain details about the different treatments available to you, their side effects and potential benefits, and predictions about their success. The checklist will also include any appropriate clinical research studies that you may want to consider participating in. (Clinical trials are discussed in Chapter 8.)

You may want to contact the American Cancer Society or the National Cancer Institute's "Physicians Data Query" (PDQ) dur-

Patient's Checklist

Your name and address:

Your primary doctor's name and specialty:

The names of other doctors involved in your care:

Diagnosis

Type of tumor and tumor site:

Clinical Staging Studies

Clinical stage:

Blood tests:

Imaging studies:

Pathological Staging Studies

Pathological stage:

Additional biopsies:

Treatment Options

*Surgery

Extent of procedure and length of hospitalization:

Side effects:

Expected results:

*Radiation therapy

Region of the body to be treated:

Duration of treatment:

Side effects:

Expected results:

*Systemic therapy

Drugs or agents to be used or considered:

Treatment schedule:

Hospitalization required?

Side effects:

Expected results:

Combination therapy

Sequence if this option is used:

Clinical trial

Type of treatment:

Summary of Treatment Options

Final Plan

---

ing your information-gathering period (see pages 20–22 for specific information about these and other organizations). In addition to these formal sources, information is increasingly available on the Internet. Use a great deal of caution here, however, because much of the information on the Internet has not been officially reviewed or edited, and some "information" may actually be advertisements for a particular doctor's practice or treatment. The information from other patients in the chat rooms or bulletin boards may be interesting, but it may not apply to your specific disease or situation.

Some of the treatments advertised on the Internet are alternative, complementary, or unproven treatments. In the introduction to this book I provided some guidelines for thinking about these treatments. Let me say here that, although we all want a good result of treatment, for some people with cancer, no really effective therapy is available. For these people, unconventional treatments can be especially tempting. As noted earlier, some unconventional treatments can be helpful or at least do no harm if used along with conventional therapies. But some of these therapies may be harmful, especially if they are substituted for conventional treatment. Others can seriously compromise the quality of a patient's

Sources of Information and Assistance for Patients

American Cancer Society (ACS). A national organization with local chapters which helps in the fight against cancer, the ACS is involved in a variety of activities, including research, patient and public education, and prevention. The national office is in Atlanta, Georgia, and divisional offices are located in most major cities throughout the United States: New York, Chicago, and San Francisco, for example. The ACS is a great source of information and assistance. See www.cancer.org.

Internet. A tremendous amount of information can be found on the Internet, including governmental agencies, private agencies, patient advocacy and support groups, university cancer centers, private hospitals and physicians, bulletin boards for patient-physician discussions, and advertisements for products. This information should be used carefully, since much of it has not been officially reviewed or edited and some of the "information" may be advertisements for individual physicians' practices or treatments.

National Cancer Institute (NCI). One of the twenty institutes of the National Institutes of Health, the NCI has the mission of fighting cancer in numerous ways, including through basic science, clinical science, prevention, screening, epidemiology, and information services. With its main offices located in Bethesda, Maryland, the NCI supports research programs throughout the United States and in other countries as well. The NCI is funded by the federal government as part of the Department of Health and Human Services (DHHS). The use of its funds is carefully reviewed by experts. Research grants are awarded to investigators in a peer-review system designed to ensure that the highest quality work is done. See www.nci.nih.gov.

National Coalition for Cancer Survivorship (NCCS). A private organization with an interest in issues related to cancer survivorship and to cancer care in general. The research issues include cancer screening, prevention, and treatment. Issues facing long-term survivors include possible work discrimination and difficulties in obtaining insurance. The NCCS is located at 1010 Wayne Avenue, Suite 200, Silver

Spring, Maryland 20910 (telephone 301-650-9127). See www.cancer advocacy.org.

National Comprehensive Cancer Network (NCCN). Develops treatment guidelines and information for patients and professionals. See www.nccn.org.

National Institutes of Health (NIH). The NIH consists of twenty institutes, including the NCI, which are part of the federal government's Department of Health and Human Services. The NIH is located in Bethesda, Maryland. Each institute is devoted to a different disease: in addition to the National Cancer Institute, there are the National Heart, Lung, and Blood Institute, the National Institute of Allergy and Infectious Diseases, and the National Institute of Mental Health, and others. See www.nih.gov.

Office of Cancer Complementary and Alternative Medicine (OCCAM), National Cancer Institute (NCI), and National Center for Complementary and Alternative Medicine (NCCAM), NIH. The OCCAM was established to coordinate and enhance activities of the NCI in complementary and alternative medicine (CAM) research as it relates to the prevention, diagnosis, and treatment of cancer, cancer-related symptoms, and side effects of conventional cancer treatment. See www.cancer.gov/cam/. For general information about complementary and alternative medicine, contact the National Center for Complementary and Alternative Medicine (NCCAM) Clearinghouse at 1-888-NIH-NCAM (1-888-644-6226) or see nccam.nih.gov.

Patient Advocacy Groups. Many groups have been formed which focus on specific cancers, such as breast cancer and prostate cancer. These groups are involved in a wide range of activities, including patient information, political lobbying, and support for people with cancer. The names of these groups are available at most cancer centers and on the Internet.

Physicians Data Query (PDQ). A computerized data base with an editorial board of cancer experts. Data are available to medical libraries, individual institutions, and various commercial cancer information services. The sections containing treatment recommendations list the range of acceptable treatments as well as treatments that require further testing. PDQ will not give you any specific recommendations regarding your treatment and certainly isn't intended to replace an expert physician. However, the background information about the cancer and the list of treatment and research options can be extremely helpful and reassuring. The service is located in Bethesda, Maryland, at the National Cancer Institute and can be contacted by telephone at 1-800/4CANCER (1-800-422-6237) or reached on the NCI Web site at www.nci.nih.gov.

---

remaining time. Again, it's a good idea to discuss such treatments with your doctor.

Personal Steps in Diagnosis and Treatment

You will need to consider all kinds of personal matters while you are deciding which treatment will be best for you. The medical information you gather during this period will not only help you make decisions about treatment, but it will also help you plan your time wisely. The answers to the questions in the preceding section ("Gather Information about Treatment Options") will provide a great deal of useful information to help you make plans. Treatments usually take a few months (and some take the better part of a year), so there will be time during the treatment to make additional adjustments in your life.

During this difficult time, it may be hard for you to manage your thoughts and emotions, which at times can be overwhelming. When you can, however, it is a good idea to think about how to structure your life in a way that will make it easier for you to cope with treatment. For example, you might make a list of the tasks you need to accomplish. In addition to medical matters, this list should include personal, work-related, financial, and legal matters that need to be handled. Setting priorities and taking care of important family and business matters will give you peace of mind, make you feel more productive, and give you a greater sense of control over what everyone agrees is a difficult situation.

You might also consider making a second list of things you like to do but haven't gotten around to doing: spending time with a friend or family member, taking a few days away at a peaceful spot, taking a ferry ride on a sunny day, or spending some time in the tranquility of nature. Although you may have to postpone doing some of the things on this second list—such as visiting relatives in another part of the country or taking a trip abroad—until you have begun or even completed treatment, having something to look forward to can be extremely important.

Discuss Treatment Options with Your Doctors

While you are working through medical and personal matters, you need to have ongoing discussions with the doctor or doctors who will be involved in your decision making and treatment. A large amount of information will be coming your way, and absorbing all the facts is difficult under the best of circumstances. It is even more difficult when experiencing the anxiety and stress associated with a major illness.

I have my own "Rule of Ten Percent," which holds that most people comprehend and remember only about one-tenth of the information they receive during a single visit with their doctors. Attending carefully to the steps in figure 1.1 and gathering and recording information in the Patient's Checklist will help you understand much more during each visit with your doctor. And it will have the added advantage of showing you what you *don't* know or understand, so you can ask more questions and seek additional information.

Throughout this process, it is important to touch base periodically with your primary doctors and with nurses, technologists, social workers, and other members of the health care team. It often is helpful to review with them the information you have gathered, to be sure that you understand it fully. Discuss the options with your health care providers. Then you might think about the options again and have another discussion, with the same individual or with someone else on the health care team.

Some people move through this process quickly, and before

long they decide what treatment option is best for them. Other people need to spend several days or longer just thinking before they can begin to make a decision.

Select the Most Appropriate Treatment

The discussion and selection process takes serious thought, but the time comes when you must make a decision about treatment. With the checklist in front of you, you and your family can review the pros and cons of each treatment option. At this point, you have digested the information about your options, you have planned your life as well as possible, and you have had a number of conversations with your doctors and other members of the health care team. Along the way, and especially when you reach the point of making a decision, it is usually a good idea to involve family members or friends, who can be extremely helpful by providing additional sets of ears, by remembering things you may have forgotten, and by serving as sounding boards.

You and your doctor will have reviewed the benefits of the different treatments to be certain that you have realistic expectations concerning what the different treatments will do for you. You will have a good understanding of the "costs" of treatment, including side effects, the time involved, the degree to which treatment will disrupt your personal life, and, possibly, the financial costs involved. After all these discussions with doctors and family and friends, you may feel that you have reached a "final" decision about treatment. But, even then, additional evaluation and discussion with your doctor may be necessary. Let me provide you with an example.

Paul R. is 68 years old and has prostate cancer. Although Paul's doctor was not able to detect the tumor during a physical examination, the results of blood tests, imaging studies, and a biopsy have indicated that Paul does have a tumor and that both sides of his prostate gland are affected. Under the circumstances, the chance that the tumor can be completely removed with surgery is fifty-fifty at best. Paul has already consulted a surgeon (a urologist), a radiation oncologist, and a medical oncologist.

After filling in the checklist and discussing the situation with his wife and children, Paul is inclined to undergo the surgery and "get it over with." However, he is understandably concerned about the recovery period and some of the potential long-term side effects of surgery, such as loss of urinary control (which rarely occurs) and loss of sexual function (which commonly occurs). He knows that radiation therapy is also effective in treating his cancer, but he is concerned because that course of treatment takes seven weeks and the long-term side effects include potential injury to his rectum (which rarely occurs) and loss of sexual function (which occurs at about the same rate as that caused by surgery).

During a discussion with his doctor, Paul says he prefers surgery. The doctor points out that the long-term cure rates and the percentage risks of serious side effects with surgery and radiation therapy are approximately equal. However, the major side effect of each treatment differs — urinary leakage for surgery and rectal irritation for radiotherapy. The doctor also points out that the features of the tumor mean that there is a fifty-fifty chance that Paul would need radiation therapy after surgery, because the surgeon might not be able to remove all the tumor cells at the margins of the gland. Finally, the doctor tells Paul that new treatments are available for men who experience the loss of sexual function after either treatment.

After some more thought, Paul might say, "What the heck. I'll take my chances with the surgery," or "Well, since there is a good chance I may need radiation therapy anyway, why don't I just take the radiation treatment and skip the operation?" Paul knows for certain that either treatment is appropriate, and he can move forward because he has clear and realistic expectations.

Complete the Treatment

Many patients find that the decision-making period is the most difficult one. Although there is no denying that the duration and intensity of treatment can make the treatment period difficult, too, many people find that, once treatment begins, things go easier, because they have clearly defined goals and mileposts and can continue working on their personal issues. Many patients say that dealing with personal matters and setting new priorities have enriched their lives and personal relationships.

Make Regular Follow-up Visits

To achieve a successful "reentry" into life's routine after treatment, and to check whether the treatment has been successful over the long term, requires a careful follow-up plan. You will need to make regular follow-up visits to the cancer specialists who treated you. Your family doctor may not be familiar with the long-term benefits and side effects of your cancer treatment, but you will consult him or her for routine health problems such as the flu or for immunizations before you take a trip abroad.

Through careful physical examinations, laboratory tests, and imaging studies, the specialists along with your primary doctor will determine the ongoing success of your treatment and investigate any long-term effects. The information obtained during follow-up visits is essential, not only to prevent problems or treat problems that may arise but also to develop better treatments for future patients. As time goes by and you are doing well, the follow-up visits will become less frequent.

It may surprise you to hear that the end of treatment also requires a period of adjustment. Throughout the treatment, you and your family have focused your energies on fighting the illness. Returning to a more normal routine after treatment often requires people to refocus their energies on regaining their physical strength and dealing with mundane matters that may seem less important than they once were.

Now that you have a "bird's-eye view" of the road ahead, we can turn, in Chapter 2, to an explanation of what happens in cancer on the cellular level—in the cells. The most confusing part of this explanation is the terminology. The general concepts themselves are not complicated. If you prefer, you can delay reading this explanation for now and skip ahead to Chapter 3, which describes how diagnostic tests and staging studies provide the information you will need to make decisions about treatment.

Chapter 2

Cancer:
Where Does It
Come From?

Cancer is a complex disease. To understand what cancer is, the first step is to understand how cells in the body behave normally. This is because, in essence, cancer is a disease in which cells act abnormally—they grow out of control.

Normal Cell Behavior

Cells do all kinds of things, including divide into more cells: one cell can divide into two cells, each "offspring cell" can divide into two cells, and so on. After dividing ten times, one cell produces 1,024 cells; after fifteen cell divisions, one cell has become 32,768 cells. Cell division occurs at various times and for various reasons: cells divide during the growth and development of the embryo and the fetus, for example, and when there is a need to repair an injury in the body, such as a scraped knee. Cells also divide in cancer—cancer occurs when they divide out of control.

As the human embryo develops, cells that at first were all the same type become specialized to perform specific functions. Some cells become muscle cells, and others become bone cells, blood cells, skin cells, or nerve cells. Even so, all cells in the body have the same basic structure—though each type of cell looks different under the microscope, depending on its function. Figure 2.1 shows the basic elements contained in every cell.

Some specialized cells, such as nerve cells, stop dividing when the individual's nervous system is completely mature. Others, such as blood cells and skin cells, continue to divide throughout a person's lifetime. Normal cells do not divide *randomly;* rather, they divide *only when they receive a signal telling them to do so.*

How Do Cells Communicate?

Cells don't do what they do alone. That is, they don't carry out their functions in isolation from what's going on around them. Not only are they in physical contact with neighboring cells, but they communicate with their neighbors as well.

One way cells communicate is with molecules called hormones, growth factors, and cytokines. All cells have some type of signaling molecules. Growth factors released from one cell can travel to an adjacent or neighboring cell, or they can travel through the bloodstream to cells in distant parts of the body. Once a growth factor or cytokine reaches another cell, it binds onto appropriate receptors on that other cell's surface in a way that resembles placing a key in a lock, as shown at the top of figure 2.1. Some of the new molecular-targeted therapies are aimed at these receptors. These therapies are discussed further in Chapter 7.

Control of Normal Cell Behavior

The behavior of every cell in the body is controlled by a highly complex molecule called *DNA* (for *deoxyribonucleic acid*), which is situated in the cell nucleus and serves as the cell's "brain." The DNA is the blueprint for everything the cell does. In a human cell, the DNA is arranged in 46 sections called *chromosomes*, which are arranged in pairs, 23 chromosomes from each parent. The chromosome pairs can be arranged in a specific order (called a *karyotype*) according to their size and shape. One of these pairs of chromosomes determines a person's sex: males have one X chromosome and one Y (XY) chromosome, whereas females have two X chromosomes (XX). Other chromosomes contain genes that determine different things about the person: height, hair color, eye color, and so on.

Together, the 46 chromosomes contain approximately 30,000 genes. (A *gene* is a segment of DNA that determines the structure of a protein.) Each gene occupies a specific location on a chromo-

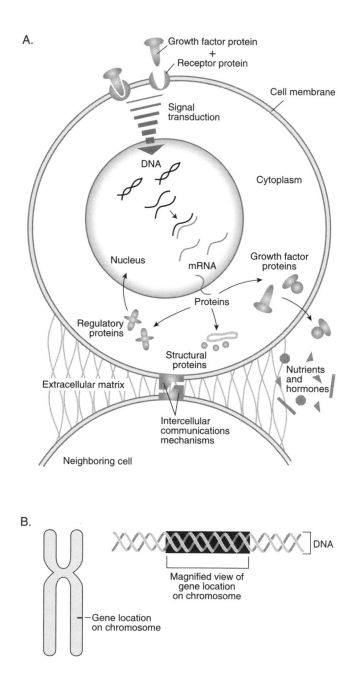

A.

Growth factor protein
+
Receptor protein

Cell membrane

Signal transduction

DNA

Cytoplasm

Nucleus

mRNA

Growth factor proteins

Regulatory proteins

Proteins

Structural proteins

Extracellular matrix

Nutrients and hormones

Intercellular communications mechanisms

Neighboring cell

B.

DNA

Magnified view of gene location on chromosome

Gene location on chromosome

some. Like the chromosomes, the genes are arranged in pairs—one gene from the mother, the other from the father. Each pair of genes is called a pair of *alleles*. When both alleles in the pair produce the same protein, they are said to be *homozygous* (the same). When each allele in the pair produces a slightly different protein, the two alleles are said to be *heterozygous* (different). A wide range of possible alleles exists, so that, except for identical twins, the proteins on the surface of each individual person's cells are different from those on the surface of the cells of every other person. That is why it is difficult to transplant organs or tissue from one person to another—even when the match is close, it's not *identical*, except in identical twins.

Through a number of biochemical steps, each gene tells a cell to make a different protein. Some genes instruct the cell to manufacture structural proteins, which serve as building blocks. Other genes tell the cell to produce hormones, growth factors, or cytokines, which (as noted above) exit the cell and communicate with other cells. Still other genes tell the cell to produce regulatory proteins that control the function of other proteins or tell other genes when to turn "on" or "off." When a gene is turned *on,* it manufactures another complex molecule called *RNA* (ribonucleic *acid*), which contains all the information the cell needs to make new

---

Fig. 2.1. Diagram of a cell (opposite)

A. The "brain" of a cell is the nucleus, which contains a molecule called DNA. The DNA is the blueprint from which the cell makes proteins. DNA is organized into chromosomes, which are subdivided into genes. RNA is made from the DNA blueprint, and proteins are made from the RNA blueprint. There are three basic classes of proteins. Regulatory proteins help control the cell's function, structural proteins are building blocks, and growth factors are molecules by which a cell communicates with its neighbors. The behavior of a cell is determined by its neighborhood, including the structure to which it is attached (called extracellular matrix), the neighboring cells, and the nutrients, hormones, and growth factors that are near the cell (in the microenvironment).

B. A gene is a segment of DNA. There are about 30,000 genes in a human cell, located on 23 pairs of chromosomes.

proteins. This *messenger RNA* (mRNA) is then transported into the cell's cytoplasm—the material surrounding the nucleus—where it directs the manufacture of a new protein.

The functions of RNA are much more complex than once thought. By a process called *RNA interference* (*RNAi*), genes can be regulated so that small pieces of RNA can actually help turn genes on and off. Furthermore, the proteins that normally surround the DNA, called *histones,* are also involved in silencing genes. Enzymes that change the histones (by processes called *methylation* and *acetylation*) can also determine which genes are on and off. Because they change the function of genes but do not change the actual structure of the DNA bases, these proteins aand enzymes are called *epigenetic modifiers.* This new knowledge is opening up exciting areas of research including novel strategies to regulate cancer cells.

A digression is called for here to explain the concept of homozygous and heterozygous as well as dominant and recessive traits. In heredity, there are two types of traits: dominant and recessive. Let's use eye color as an example. The gene for brown eyes (B) is dominant, and the gene for blue eyes (b) is recessive. If both parents are homozygous for brown eyes—that is, they have two B genes (BB) in their "eye-color" alleles, all their children will have brown eyes. If both parents are homozygous for blue eyes—they have two b genes (bb) in their "eye-color" alleles—all their children will have blue eyes. If one parent is homozygous for brown eyes (BB) and the other parent is heterozygous for eye color (Bb), all their children (who will have either BB or Bb genes) will still have brown eyes, because B is dominant. However, if both parents are heterozygous (Bb) for eye color, the children can be BB, Bb, bB, or bb. Thus, each child born to this couple has a one in four chance of having blue eyes (bb). (Because the gene for brown eyes is dominant, someone with Bb or bB genes in their "eye-color" alleles will still have brown eyes, but such a person may have offspring with blue eyes, depending upon the other parent's genes, as in the example above.)

The concepts of homozygosity and heterozygosity and of dominant and recessive traits are discussed in more detail in Appendix A. To indicate the importance of these concepts, let's say that G is a control gene needed to keep a cellular process in check. As long as there is one copy of G, then the cell behaves normally, so that GG or Gg will be fine, but gg may be a problem as both G genes are lost. But, if a person is Gx (x indicates no gene is present) and the G allele is lost completely by a mutation, the cell becomes xx and may not function normally. This process of Gx to xx can occur in the development of cancer, and is called the loss of heterozygosity, which is abbreviated as LOH.

How Normal Cells Divide

Cells divide only when they receive the proper signals from inside the cell, from growth factors that circulate in the bloodstream or from a cell they are in direct contact with. For example, if a person loses blood, a growth factor called *erythropoietin,* which is produced in the kidneys, circulates in the bloodstream and tells the bone marrow to manufacture more blood cells. Growth factors that come from outside the cell can transmit a message by binding to the appropriate receptor on the cell surface (the key and lock again), triggering a signaling system that activates a specific gene in the cell's nucleus. Other signals generated within the cell itself can use the signaling systems to activate a gene.

When a cell receives the message to divide, it goes through the cell cycle illustrated in figure 2.2. When the cell is at rest, it is said to be at G_0 (or Gap-zero). At this rest stage, no activity is visible under the microscope. When the cell receives the proper signals, it prepares to divide by entering the G_1 (or Gap-1) phase. It then enters the S (synthesis) phase, during which the cell's DNA makes an exact copy of itself—a process called *replication.* (The S-phase can be observed under the microscope.) The cell then enters a temporary resting phase (the G_2 phase) while it prepares to divide. Finally, the cell enters the M (*mitosis*) phase and becomes two cells. If all goes well, both "offspring cells" contain exact duplicates of all the genetic material contained in the parent cell's nucleus. When division is accomplished, the two offspring cells rest in the G_0 phase until they receive the signal to divide.

Checkpoints along each step of this process "look" to see

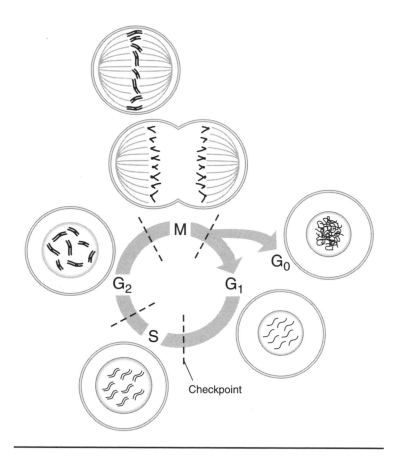

Fig. 2.2. The phases of cell division

The phases of a cell division cycle can be seen under a microscope. Most cells are in a resting phase called G_0. When they get ready to divide, they enter the cell cycle in a phase called G_1 (G stands for *gap,* as there is nothing visible to the eye, although biochemical analysis can detect changes in the cell). Next, in S (DNA synthesis), the chromosomes are duplicated so that there will be one set for each offspring cell. G_2 is the next gap in which the cell prepares to divide into two, which happens in M (mitosis). Before progressing from one phase in the cycle to another, a cell must pass through checkpoints. If damage is detected at a checkpoint, the damage is repaired, or the cell may undergo a process called *programmed cell death* (*apoptosis*), by which the defective cell is eliminated.

whether the step has been accomplished accurately. In cancer, the cell cycle may be unregulated because of defective checkpoints; that is, normal checkpoints, which are designed to regulate the cycle, are defective, and the cell cycle is not regulated as it would be if they were normal. Just the fact that the cell goes through such a cycle works to the advantage of cancer treatment, because many chemotherapeutic agents are designed to attack cells that are "in cycle," that is, cells that are dividing. Without this cycle, clearly, these agents would not be effective.

Abnormal Cell Behavior

Abnormal Cells Do Not Always Become Cancer Cells

Most abnormal cells simply deteriorate and are removed either by neighboring cells or by cells specifically designed to "clean up" debris such as deteriorating cells. This normal process of cell death and cleanup occurs at many points in life — during development of the fetus, in the maturing immune system (the body's defense against foreign substances such as bacteria and viruses), and in many other tissues as cells undergo normal turnover.

In an orderly process of cell "suicide" (called *apoptosis,* or *programmed cell death*), cells that are no longer needed are fragmented into particles and removed. If a cell develops a mutation, certain "proofreading" molecules that check the DNA or cell structure may activate the process of apoptosis and in that way get rid of the cell before it becomes a cancer. Because some cancer cells may lose the ability to undergo apoptosis, researchers are attempting to develop a way of restoring the cancer cells' ability to undergo this process, which would put a check on these cells' ability to grow out of control.

How Do Cancerous Cells Behave?

A cancer cell is a cell that grows out of control. It no longer needs signals to make it grow; it just does so on its own. No matter how a cell becomes malignant, the basic situation is that the complex processes that keep cell division in check break down, and the cell begins dividing out of control. This does not happen often, however, and so it's not easy for a cell to become malignant.

For a cell to become a cancer, a number of processes must go wrong, including those that control cell division, the cell cycle, the ability to invade surrounding tissue, the ability to metastasize to other parts of the body, and the ability to make new blood vessels.

The many processes that must take place correctly for a cell to divide properly are described above. For one thing, the DNA must be duplicated precisely, so that each offspring cell has a complete set of the parent cell's chromosomes. The cell cycle has many checkpoints to detect damage and either repair it or initiate the cell suicide process. If one of the many checkpoints that control the process of cell division is defective, however, an abnormal cell may be allowed to divide.

In a cancer cell, several genes change (mutate) and the cell becomes defective. There are two general types of gene mutations. One type, called a *dominant mutation,* is caused by an abnormality in one gene in a pair. It is a "gain of function" mutation. An example is a mutated gene that produces a defective protein that causes a growth-factor receptor on the cell's surface to be constantly "on" when, in fact, no growth factor is present. Thus, the cell receives a constant message to divide. This dominant, gain of function gene is often called an *oncogene (onco = cancer).*

The second general type of mutation is a *recessive mutation;* this is a "loss of function" mutation. In this case, *both* genes in the pair must be damaged before the cell becomes cancerous — that is, one normal gene is enough. For example, a normal gene called p53 produces a protein that turns "off" the cell cycle and thus helps to control cell growth. This type of gene is called an *anti-oncogene* or *tumor suppressor gene.* If one p53 gene in the pair is mutated, the other gene will still be able to control the cell cycle. However, if both p53 genes are mutated, the "off" switch is lost, and cell division is no longer under control.

Thus, abnormal cell division, or cells growing out of control, can occur either *when active oncogenes are expressed* or *when tumor suppressor genes are lost.* As already indicated, for a cell to become malignant, numerous mutations are necessary. In some cases, both types of mutations—dominant and recessive—may occur.

A gene mutation may allow an already abnormal cell to invade the normal tissue where the cancer started, or to travel in the bloodstream (metastasize) to remote parts of the body, where it continues to divide. Metastases most often occur in the lymph nodes, lungs, liver, bone, and brain.

A normal gene can become damaged in different ways. A cell can become abnormal when part of a gene is lost (deleted), when part of a chromosome is rearranged and ends up in the wrong place on a chromosome (called a *translocation*), or when an extremely small defect occurs in the DNA, which results in an abnormal DNA "blueprint" and production of a defective protein. (A more detailed explanation of how these defects occur can be found in Appendix A.)

There are even more ways than this for an abnormal cell to begin dividing out of control, however. For example, a gene may be normal, but the protein it makes may not function normally because the cell contains a cancer-producing virus. Women infected with human papilloma virus have an increased risk of developing cancer of the cervix, because the human papilloma virus interferes with normal cell function. Whether a normal protein will function properly also depends on the cell's microenvironment; for example, normal cells have enough oxygen, but tumors can outgrow their blood supply. Cells in a situation where they have very low oxygen (called *hypoxia*) may not function normally.

The Normal Cells within a Tumor Can Take Part in the Development of the Cancer

The cancer cell does not live in isolation but is located within a complex environment, often called a *microenvironment*. For example, in a glandular tumor like prostate or breast cancer, which are both called *adenocarcinoma*, the cancer cell may be located next to a normal glandular cell; underlying supporting or connective tissue cells, called stromal cells; blood vessel cells; and immune cells and inflammatory cells. Glandular cells are attached, or anchored, to a protein scaffold called the *extracellular matrix* (see figure 2.1) or to a basement membrane. If a normal cell loses contact with its basement membrane it may die in a process called *anoikis* (an-o-EE-kis), which is similar to apoptosis. A property of cancer is *anchorage independence*—that is, the ability of a cell to live away from its normal anchorage attachments.

Other cells in the microenvironment such as the connective tissue, immune cells, and inflammatory cells can produce factors that stimulate the growth of the glandular and cancer cells. The presence of chronic inflammation may be an important factor in the development of cancer. For this reason, drugs that target inflammation are being studied to prevent (*chemoprevention*) or treat certain cancers, for example, colon cancer and prostate cancer.

A Cancer Cell's Behavior Depends on What Has Gone Wrong

Thus, cancer can be caused by processes that do not work properly for a variety of reasons. How a specific cancer cell behaves depends on which processes are not functioning properly. Some cancer cells simply divide and produce more cancer cells, and the tumor mass stays where it began. Other cancer cells are able to invade normal tissue, enter the bloodstream, and metastasize to a remote site in the body. It is not possible to tell how a cell will behave simply by looking at it under the microscope. There are new techniques that allow scientists to study the individual molecules (this field is called *molecular biology*). More information on this topic is provided in Appendix A.

Like all living things, cells need nourishment. This is supplied by the bloodstream, which carries nutrients to and waste products away from the cell's microenvironment. One important nutrient the bloodstream supplies to cells is oxygen, which is necessary for all living things, including cells. Cells can live for only a brief time without oxygen. For cancers to continue to grow, the cells must produce proteins called *angiogenesis factors,* which cause the growth of new blood vessels to bring the cells the oxygen and other nutrients they need to survive. A novel form of treatment called *antiangiogenic treatment* targets the tumor blood vessels. An antibody called bevacizumab (Avastin®) has been approved for clinical use, and many more drugs are under development to target developing blood vessels as well as established blood vessels.

In summary, a cancer cell has defects in normal functions which allow it to divide, invade the surrounding tissue, and spread by way of the bloodstream. The defects are the result of gene mutations abnormal protein function, or infections by viruses. In essence, cancer is not a single disease but many diseases. This makes it complicated for scientists, but it also offers many targets by which to kill the cancer cells.

Cancer and Heredity

Cancer cannot be inherited, but the *risk* of developing cancer can be. That is, the *tendency* to develop cancer runs in some families, as has been shown with the discovery of specific abnormal genes that make a woman more likely to develop breast cancer under certain conditions. The presence of genetic abnormalities doesn't mean that the disease itself is hereditary, however.

In cancers with a hereditary component, an abnormal gene is passed from parent to child. However, a cell becomes abnormal during a person's lifetime because of additional changes in the DNA such as a spontaneous gene mutation or a cancer-causing agent (*carcinogen*) in the environment. Asbestos, cigarette smoking, and some pesticides are well-known carcinogens. According to the information that is currently available, the majority of cancers appear to be the spontaneous variety rather than the inherited kind linked to predisposition.

Another extremely important point to remember is that many people who have either an inherited cancer gene or a gene that has mutated spontaneously do not develop the disease. The abnormal gene might mean a tendency to develop a cancer, but additional mutations must occur before a tumor can develop. In fact, *most cancer cells have a number of different defects in their DNA.* Thus, one abnormal gene rarely causes cancer.

Genetic Counseling

Genetic counseling is a new and rapidly evolving field that is important for parents who are concerned that they may pass a disease, such as sickle-cell anemia, cystic fibrosis, or cancer, to their children. Genetic counselors interview couples about their family histories to determine what type of disease may have occurred in relatives. For example, because some cancers, such as breast and ovarian cancer, go together, women whose relatives have developed either type of cancer at a young age may be at risk for either type of cancer. Under certain circumstances, a genetic counselor may recommend that a person have his or her genes examined in the laboratory. (Several methods used to study genes in the laboratory are described in Appendix A.) If a genetic abnormality is identified, the counselor can then discuss the potential risks for them or their children, the need for regular screening, and preventive measures. In some situations this may even involve the removal of an organ; for example, some women at risk for developing breast and ovarian cancer may have prophylactic removal of their ovaries. Obviously, this requires careful discussion with doctors and family members.

Although genetic counseling can be helpful in some cases, it also raises a number of difficult questions:

— Can something be done to prevent the cancer? If nothing can be done to prevent the cancer, can more frequent testing for the cancer, and early detection, at least make a difference in terms of treatment and recovery?

— Will the information make the person's life better or worse? That is, will worry about the possibility of developing cancer dominate the person's thoughts, so that his or her quality of life is diminished?

— Will the information be kept confidential, so that insurance companies and employers don't have access to it? (Insurance companies and employers may discriminate against a person if genetic testing indicates that he or she has inherited a tendency to develop cancer.)

Because questions such as these sometimes have unsatisfactory answers, many people, understandably, avoid genetic testing. The decision to undergo genetic testing is a difficult and personal one. It should be made only after discussion with an expert in oncology or genetic counseling.

Current Research

Scientists in many fields are involved in research on the biology of cancer. Among others, cellular biologists, molecular biologists, structural biologists, and tumor biologists; biochemists; physiologists; immunologists; oncologists; and pharmacologists have all recently contributed to fundamental knowledge about the complicated process called cancer. Their contributions are leading to the development of unique treatments. Because knowledge about the biology of cancer is growing extremely quickly, what was a dream only a few years ago is becoming a reality.

Since the early part of the 21st century, there has been rapid progress in understanding cancer biology and turning this knowledge into new treatments. Many new drugs are more specific in their targets. These targets include cell surface receptors, signaling pathways within the cell, apoptosis molecules, protein metabolism, angiogenesis factors, and many others. Scientists are now able to study the cancer cell signature using molecular biology techniques broadly called *genomics* (which studies DNA and RNA), proteomics (protein), metabolomics (biochemistry), and other "omics," as they are called. These "omics" are described in Appendix A. Using a tumor's molecular signature or molecular profile will help determine prognosis and treatment for a patient. This era of personalized medicine is rapidly emerging from research in the laboratory and from clinical trials.

It often takes many years before a discovery in the laboratory can be translated into a new treatment. One reason is the essential testing that must be performed, on laboratory animals and on humans, before a new treatment can be widely used. (Clinical tests using humans are discussed in Chapter 8.) Even though the results of current research discoveries will not be available as treatment for some time, the astounding rate at which new knowledge is being generated offers much cause for hope for the future.

Armed with this basic understanding of what goes wrong in cancer cells, we return, in the next chapter, to two of the steps in the Patient's Checklist described in Chapter 1: diagnosis and the staging studies.

Chapter 3

Diagnostic Tests and Staging Studies: Gathering Information

Cancers are named according to the organ in which they begin, and even if a cancer metastasizes to another part of the body, it keeps its original name. For example, breast cancer that has spread to the lungs is called metastatic breast cancer, not lung cancer, and prostate cancer that has spread to bone is called metastatic prostate cancer, not bone cancer.

Other names for types of cancer with which you may be familiar include *carcinoma, sarcoma,* and *lymphoma.* These, too, are names having to do with the part of the body in which the cancer started. *Carcinoma* is the general term for tumors that arise in epithelial tissues such as the skin and the lining of such organs as the uterus and lungs. (Saying that a woman has *uterine carcinoma* is the same thing as saying that she has *cancer of the uterus.*) Tumors that arise in connective tissue, such as muscle or bone, are called *sarcomas.* Brain tumors are called *gliomas,* tumors that begin in the lymph system are called *lymphomas,* and cancers that arise in bone marrow are called *leukemias.* Table 3.1 identifies these different types of cancer.

The terms *tumor, mass,* and *lump* are often used interchangeably to mean any overgrowth of tissue. Someone who has a tumor, a mass, or a lump does not necessarily have cancer, however. Many tumors do not contain cancer cells. For example, small fatty tumors called *lipomas* occur commonly in the skin. Some tumors —called *benign tumors*—can cause pain or other problems (they may interfere with normal body functions, for example), and they may need to be surgically removed. But they are not malignant.

Many people think only of cancer when they hear the word *tu-*

Table 3.1. Types of Cancer and the Tissues or Organs Involved

Type of Cancer	Tissue or Organ Where the Cancer Originates
Carcinomas	
Adenocarcinoma	Cells lining the ducts of glands or cells from glandular tissue. Cancer of the breast, lung, prostate, gastrointestinal tract, and glandular structures such as salivary glands, pancreas, and endocrine glands can be adenocarcinoma.
Carcinoma	A general term for all types of cancer beginning in epithelial tissue (which lines the surface of organs or body cavities—e.g., skin, gastrointestinal tract, bronchi, mouth).
Carcinoma in situ	An early cancer that occurs in a glandular or lining structure. Examples include the cervix, head and neck, breast, and skin. Although the cells are cancerous, they have not invaded the surrounding tissue (they have remained "in site"). Cancer in situ can be either adenocarcinoma or squamous carcinoma.
Endometrial	Uterus
Hepatoma	Liver
Non–small cell, small cell	Lung; small cell cancers can occur at other sites, e.g., cervix.
Squamous carcinoma	Cells on the surface of the body or cells that line internal structures such as the mouth, throat, bronchus, and anal canal
Transitional cell	Bladder
Germ cell tumors	Tumors arising in the testis or ovary. Seminomas and nonseminomas are two types of germ cell tumors of the testis.
Gliomas	
Glioblastoma	Brain
Astrocytoma	Brain
Leukemias	Bone marrow, the soft tissue in the center of bones where blood cells are manufactured

Table 3.1. Continued

Type of Cancer	Tissue or Organ Where the Cancer Originates
Lymphomas Hodgkin's disease Non-Hodgkin's lymphoma	Cells in the lymph system which manufacture immune cells
Melanoma	Pigmented cells, usually in the skin
Mesothelioma	Tissue lining the lung or abdominal cavity
Multiple myeloma	Antibody-producing immune cells
Sarcomas	Bone or connective tissue such as muscle
Seminomas	Germ cells in the testis or ovary

mor, and indeed many doctors refer to such growths as *lumps* for this reason — to avoid unnecessarily upsetting a patient. Whenever a tumor, mass, or lump is identified which might be either cancerous or benign, or might even just be scar tissue, a biopsy and imaging studies are usually performed to find out what's going on (see below). If the tumor is found to be malignant, then a series of staging studies are performed to find out more information. Most of the rest of this chapter is about these studies.

Screening and Diagnosis

One reason doctors recommend routine physical checkups is that abnormal lumps (tumors) may be discovered during the physical examination, and other potential malignancies may be discovered through the routine diagnostic screening tests that are done at this time. Having regular checkups and appropriate screening procedures can be helpful for certain cancers, because if a person develops cancer, the cancer is more likely to be caught early, when there are more treatment options. In addition to performing a physical examination, the family doctor may order routine screening procedures such as a Pap smear to detect cervical cancer, a blood test to detect prostate cancer, or a mammogram to detect breast cancer. New tests are being evaluated for lung cancer screening (spiral CT scans).

A person's age and family history generally determine the frequency with which routine screening tests are performed. Studies of cancer susceptibility genes were discussed in Chapter 2. When results of any screening test are abnormal, the results must be interpreted carefully. Screening tests cannot always definitively identify cancer; they may only indicate that there's a need for more frequent screening tests. For example, the results of a Pap smear may indicate the presence of abnormal cells in the cervix. From experience, the pathologist and the gynecologist know that over time these cells *may* become cancer cells—or they may not. In such a case, the gynecologist would follow the situation carefully, probably advising the woman to have more frequent Pap smears. On the other hand, the results of a Pap smear might indicate that cancer cells are present, in which case staging studies or a biopsy needs to be performed.

Many people visit a doctor when they have symptoms, of course, and some of these symptoms may indicate the possibility of cancer—a lump in the breast, for example, or a change in the color or size of a mole, or severe headaches in a person who has no history of migraines. When a doctor determines that a person's symptoms might be due to cancer, or if something suggests cancer during routine examination and screening tests, the diagnosis is usually established with a biopsy—the surgical removal of a small piece of tissue. If the tissue contains cancer cells, the next step is to determine the "stage" of the cancer using one of the staging systems described below.

Three very important points: Good screening procedures have not yet been developed for all types of cancer, and even when good screening is done, some cancers will not necessarily be detected at an early stage. Abnormalities detected on screening studies are *not* necessarily cancer.

Staging Systems

Staging systems are used to indicate the extent of a person's cancer, the treatment regimen that is appropriate, and the prognosis. The treatments recommended by oncologists usually depend on the clinical (observed) changes and the pathological (structural and functional) changes that characterize a specific type of cancer. Information from the molecular signature or profile of the tumor is now being used to help guide treatment (see Chapter 2 and Appendix A). (The natural history of a tumor also plays a role in determining treatment; this important factor is discussed later in this chapter.) People with more advanced disease usually require more aggressive treatment, but if they receive the proper treatment, their prognosis may be as good as that of people with a less advanced stage of the same disease.

Some staging systems use numbers (1, 2, 3, or 4) to identify the stage of a cancer. Others rely on Roman numerals (I, II, III, or IV), and still others use letters (A, B, C, or D). There may be a substage, such as A1 or A2. In all staging systems, the higher the number or letter, the greater the amount of the body involved in the cancer. For instance, Stage I breast cancer is a small tumor (about 1 inch or less in diameter) with no lymph nodes involved. Stage II disease means that the tumor is between 2 and 5 centimeters in diameter (about 1 or 2 inches) in the breast, that lymph nodes are involved, or both. Stage III disease means that the tumor is larger than 5 centimeters (2 inches or more) in diameter, and Stage IV disease means that the tumor involves multiple organs.

With staging systems that are more complicated (but very useful), various parts of the cancer are graded separately. Most common is the "TNM system," in which T refers to the size of the primary tumor, N indicates whether lymph nodes are involved, and M indicates whether the cancer has metastasized to another part of the body. For example, the stage of a tumor in the breast which is between 2 and 5 centimeters in diameter and involves one lymph node but no other parts of the body would be T2N1M0. A prostate cancer involving both sides of the gland and invading the surrounding tissue but with no involvement of the lymph nodes or distant metastases would be staged T3N0M0. (It is staged T3 because it is no longer confined to the prostate.) A lung cancer that is 4 centimeters in diameter, with regional lymph nodes involved and distant bone metastases, would be staged T2N2M1 (T2 because it is greater than 2 centimeters but not invading other structures in the chest; N2 because it involves lymph nodes in the chest somewhat near the tumor; and M1 because it has metastasized to bones). It's easy to see that this system provides more information, and more specific information, and therefore is useful for doctors to use when communicating with each other and determining the proper course of treatment.

Clinical Staging

The clinical stage of a cancer can be determined with a physical examination, blood tests, and imaging studies. These steps often provide very useful information about the stage of a cancer — that is, its extent, the appropriate treatment, and the prognosis. In some instances, nothing else is required; in other instances, a biopsy of the tissue in addition to a biopsy of the tumor mass may be necessary.

Physical Examination

Most people are familiar with what goes on during a routine physical examination. In a physical examination for clinical staging of cancer, your doctor checks you over in the same way but may perform additional procedures such as a *bronchoscopy* to look into your lungs or an *endoscopy* to examine the inside of your stomach or intestines.

Blood Tests

The blood tests used for clinical staging usually include routine blood counts, blood chemistries, and in some instances the evaluation of biomarkers, discussed later in this chapter. To obtain a blood count, a specific quantity of a person's blood is withdrawn, and the numbers of red and white cells and platelets in the blood sample are counted. If the number of red blood cells is too low, the person is anemic. If the white cell count is too low, it means that the person's ability to fight infection is compromised. And if the platelet count is too low, the person's blood can't clot properly. This test is often called a *complete blood count* (or CBC). Because the CBCs of most patients are normal before treatment begins, this information serves as an important *baseline* (that is, the effect of treatment on the body can be monitored by comparing later CBCs with this, the first one). Blood chemistry tests (also performed on blood that has been withdrawn from the person) measure whether the liver, kidneys, and other organs are functioning properly.

Other blood tests can detect cell products that may indicate the presence of a cancer. These cell products in the blood are called *markers* or *biomarkers*. Biomarkers are normally present in the blood in small amounts. When the amount of a particular biomarker is greater than normal, however, a cancer may be present. Because only some cancers produce these biomarkers, and because elevated levels do not necessarily indicate the presence of a tumor, the results must be carefully evaluated by a doctor. (*Note:* Tests for biomarkers are also done during the course of treatment, to determine whether tumor cells are still present.)

The following are some of the common tumor markers found in the blood when cancer is present. New biomarkers are constantly being discovered, including protein patterns (*proteomics;* see Appendix A).

— CEA (carcinoembryonic antigen) suggests lung, gastrointestinal, and breast cancer
— CA 19-9 suggests gastrointestinal cancer
— AFP (alpha-fetoprotein) and beta-HCG (human chorionic gonadotropin) suggest a germ-cell tumor of the testis or ovary
— OC-125 suggests ovarian cancer
— PSA (prostate specific antigen) suggests prostate cancer

Using tumor biomarkers to screen for cancer is controversial for two reasons: First, what criteria should determine which people should be screened? And, second, what should be done with the information obtained? Will having the information that an older individual has a small cancer, for example, lead to unnecessary anxiety for the individual, who would otherwise never be bothered by the cancer in his or her lifetime? Or will it lead to unnecessary treatment? To be useful, a screening test must accurately identify which patients need treatment, and, of course, there is no good reason to screen unless effective treatments exist for the specific disease. Answering questions about when and how to use screening tests is not always easy, but it seems likely that in the future, as we develop a better understanding of the significance of the different test results, we will be able to make even better decisions about who should be tested and when to test, when to treat, and when to hold off on treatment until there is an indication that treatment is necessary.

Consider one example of widespread screening for tumor markers: the PSA screening test for prostate cancer. The effect of the widespread use of this test has been to bring many men to the attention of the health care system who were unaware that they had the disease. Take, for example, Jim K., whose case is described in Chapter 9. A slightly elevated amount of PSA in Jim's blood led to a series of tests indicating that Jim did indeed have a tiny cancer in his prostate gland. Small tumors such as Jim's do not necessarily cause problems, and if they do, it may not be for another 10 or more years. To determine whether Jim needs treatment for the tumor in his prostate gland, his oncologist must estimate how the tumor is likely to behave, and he must take into account Jim's life expectancy. If Jim were 90 years old rather than 68, he would probably not need treatment, since the tumor is likely to grow only slowly and would be unlikely to cause symptoms or shorten life. Many such "indolent" tumors are simply observed and are treated only if they show signs of progressing. This is called watchful waiting or deferred therapy. Jim is relatively young, however, and he is healthy and active, so he and his oncologist determine that treating the cancer is going to have the best outcome for Jim.

Imaging Studies

A variety of diagnostic imaging studies can be used to determine the site of a cancer. (*Note:* Imaging studies are also used to determine how a tumor has responded to treatment, so they are done during and after treatment as well as before treatment.) These studies include x-rays, computerized tomographic (CT) scans, magnetic resonance imaging (MRI), ultrasonography, nuclear medicine scans, and positron emission tomographic (PET) scans. With the exception of the internal probe that may be used in ultrasonography and in some MRI procedures, nothing is inserted in the patient in these tests (they are not *invasive* tests), but sometimes a contrast material is injected into the patient's vein shortly before the imaging study is performed. Occasionally, contrast material can be taken by mouth.

Here's how imaging studies might be used to provide staging information about a patient with breast cancer. In the second case study described in Chapter 9, a mammogram confirmed that 47-year-old Jane S. had a small lump in her right breast. The results of a chest x-ray and bone scan were normal, indicating that the cancer had not spread beyond the breast. Her tumor was surgically removed and was found to be approximately 2.5 centimeters (about 1 inch) in diameter. It was assigned a clinical stage (CS) of IIA or T2N0M0 because the staging studies to that point indicated that no lymph nodes or other areas of the body were involved. The nodes that train the tumor were sampled by a technique called *sentinel node biopsy,* now commonly used for staging a number of different cancers. This biopsy involves injecting a small amount of dye or radioactive tracer near the tumor, tracking which lymph nodes it goes to, and then removing those specific lymph nodes (the sentinel nodes) for further analysis.

In an MRI study, a large magnet and radio waves make use of the magnetic properties of molecules to produce images of internal tissues as the patient lies in a long tunnel listening to the loud sounds of the working machine. In ultrasonography, images of internal tissues are produced by bouncing sound waves off internal body structures, much as a ship's sonar bounces sound waves off submarines beneath the surface of the water in order to identify what kind of submarine it is. The images are produced when an ultrasonographic probe is either moved slowly across the person's skin or inserted into the esophagus, rectum, or vagina. In a CT scan, a portion of the body is imaged as the patient lies in a ring in which the x-ray tube moves.

Patients who undergo a PET scan or a regular nuclear medicine scan are injected with radioactive elements called *isotopes,* and the tissues are then examined with a specialized camera. Different isotopes are required depending on the type of tissue scanned — bone, liver, or lung, for example. The radioactive material poses little danger to patients or family members, because it usually lasts for only a few hours or a day, it decays to the point where there is essentially no radiation left, and the minute amount of radioactivity that remains is eliminated in the urine or feces.

Pathological Staging

Occasionally, surgery or another procedure is performed to obtain additional tissue that may be involved with a tumor. For example, surgery may be used to remove lymph nodes or explore the abdominal organs, and other procedures may be used to obtain a sample of bone marrow or spinal fluid. These studies should be performed only if the information obtained that way is necessary to determine which treatment will be best.

Because breast cancer often involves the lymph nodes, many women who have breast cancer undergo additional biopsies. For example, after Jane S.'s tumor was removed, the surgeon removed a sample of lymph nodes from her right armpit. When the pathologist examined the lymph tissue under a high-powered microscope, he found that one lymph node was cancerous. As a result, the stage of Jane's cancer was changed from CS IIA (clinical stage) to pathological stage (PS) IIB (T2N1M0), and her treatment options were revised accordingly.

When determining the tumor type, pathologists use a variety of techniques. Under the normal light microscope, they examine the tumor's overall structure. When necessary, using an electron microscope, they examine the individual cancer cells. Pathologists can also employ specific techniques to detect proteins in or on the cell (called *immunohistochemical studies,* these are described in more detail below). Under some circumstances, so that a more precise diagnosis can be made, a surgeon may have to repeat a biopsy to obtain additional tissues just for these pathological and molecular studies (described in Appendix A).

Tumor Grading Systems

Pathologists assign a pathological grade to a tumor according to how malignant the tissue looks under the microscope. The grade may be an important factor when estimating a person's prognosis and determining the optimal treatment. Tumor grades can be expressed in words or by a number. One set of terms consists of *well differentiated, moderately differentiated,* or *poorly differentiated.* The organ of origin of well-differentiated tumors can be readily identified, because the tumor cells resemble normal cells, whereas identifying the organ of origin of poorly differentiated cells can be difficult. When tumors are graded by number (1 through 4), a Grade-1 tumor has a better natural history (see below) than a Grade-4 tumor does. Betty, in the example below, had a well-differentiated tumor.

A tumor that has the tendency to invade into the small blood or lymph vessels or to invade into the surrounding tissue is more aggressive and would likely require a different treatment. The pathologist will look for lymphatic vessel invasion (LVI) or capillary (blood vessel) invasion (vascular invasion). Some new research suggests that tumors that make many new blood vessels (called microvessel density) have a greater tendency to produce metastases. The pathologist, therefore, might also estimate microvessel density as part of a study. Before making cut sections of the tissue (surgical specimen) that the surgeon has removed, the pathologist may put ink on all the margins. When she looks under the microscope, the pathologist can then tell if tumor cells reached the margin of the specimen. This would be a positive margin. There are new experimental approaches using molecular biology techniques to try to see if there are cells left behind which cannot be

seen by the surgeon or even by the pathologist under the microscope. The surgeon will give the pathologist a very small sample
of the normal tissue that surrounds the tumor, and then special
laboratory tests are done to see if cells can be detected which are
too few in number to be seen under the microscope.

> During a routine annual physical examination, it was discov-
> ered that Betty had a half-inch lump in her thyroid. She under-
> went a procedure called a *fine needle aspirate (FNA)* of her thy-
> roid to remove tissue for examination under the microscope.
> The cells in the tissue looked almost exactly like normal thy-
> roid cells, but the nuclei were a little too big. A thyroid sur-
> geon removed part of the thyroid gland and, indeed, found a
> small cancer that looked very much like normal thyroid. Betty
> underwent additional treatment with radioactive iodine and
> then was put on thyroid hormone pills to supply the thyroid
> hormone that her own thyroid would no longer be able to pro-
> duce. She is cured of her thyroid cancer.

Prostate cancer is graded according to the Gleason system,
which ranges from grade 2 to grade 10. According to this system,
the Gleason grade of Jim K.'s cancer was 6. Generally, men whose
tumors are in the lowest grades (2 to 6) do well, whereas a prostate cancer graded 8 to 10 is highly likely to have metastasized
cancer beyond the prostate gland. Men with tumors graded 7 are
in-between.

How Pathologists Examine Tissue
Histological Studies

At the time of an initial biopsy, a pathologist can provide the surgeon with preliminary information by quickly freezing a sample
of the tissue, cutting a thin slice, staining it, and examining its
structural (histological) characteristics under a microscope. As
a result of this preliminary information, the surgeon will know
whether to remove the remaining tumor and how much tissue at
the margins of the tumor also need to be removed.

To obtain a more accurate diagnosis, the tissue removed during the biopsy is embedded in a block of paraffin, sliced into sections, stained, and examined under the microscope. This process usually takes a few days, and specific immunologic and molecular studies may take a week or more.

Immunologic studies. As described in Chapter 2, all cells have a variety of proteins on their surface. Some of these proteins are called *lineage specific* because all cells of the same type have similar proteins. For example, certain proteins on the surface of lymph cells differ from those on the surface of cells lining the stomach. Using substances called *monoclonal antibodies* which are tagged with a fluorescent substance, pathologists can study a section of tissue under the microscope and, by identifying the proteins on the cells' surface, determine the type of cell involved. This procedure, called *immunohistochemistry,* is particularly useful when cancer cells are poorly differentiated or when the specific type of cancer must be identified, as with lymphomas.

Molecular studies. To diagnose some cancers, it may be necessary for the pathologist to identify abnormalities in the genes themselves, using molecular biology techniques. The chromosomes in a cancer cell can also be isolated and studied in the laboratory. Certain cancers have specific chromosomal abnormalities. (These complex procedures are described in Appendix A.)

Lumbar Punctures

Lumbar puncture is performed in order to stage certain leukemias and lymphomas. For this procedure, after the patient receives a local anesthetic, a needle is inserted into the lumbar sac in the lower back, and a sample of spinal fluid is withdrawn. This procedure is relatively safe because the spinal cord ends above the lumbar sac (so there is little or no danger of injuring the cord). Because the spinal fluid circulates freely between the brain, the spinal cord, and the lumbar sac, lumbar punctures can also be used to inject drugs into the central nervous system to prevent disease or to administer chemotherapy to the brain.

Natural History of a Tumor

In addition to information gathered from the staging studies, when deciding on a course of treatment to recommend, the oncologist takes into account how a specific type of cancer usually behaves. This behavior, called the *natural history of a tumor,* is an important factor in selecting the appropriate treatment regimen for a specific cancer. Some cancers are extremely aggressive: they invade the surrounding tissue and spread quickly throughout the body. Others remain stable for many years without treatment (these "indolent" cancers include some extremely early prostate cancers, chronic leukemias, and low-grade lymphomas). In considering the natural history of the tumor in order to choose treatment, the oncologist attempts to determine, as accurately as possible, the answers to these questions:

— How is the cancer likely to behave if it is not treated?
— How long will it be before the patient develops symptoms?
— Is the cancer likely to spread and, if so, to what organs?
— Will the disease be cured by a local treatment?
— Will the patient require more surgery?
— Will the cancer cells be killed by radiation therapy or chemotherapy, or will they be resistant to these treatments?
— Will a combination of treatments be best?
— Should an experimental treatment be recommended?

Despite what we know about the natural history of a specific kind of cancer, it is not possible to answer many of these questions precisely for a specific individual, and what we know about the natural history of a cancer may not hold true for a specific individual. Nevertheless, the natural history of the cancer forms a very important part of the "big picture" when oncologists select treatments.

Prognosis

Your prognosis—how your cancer is likely to respond to treatment—is determined by the type of cancer you have as well as a variety of other factors. Keep in mind that a prognosis is only an estimate of how a person will do as a result of treatment (see Chapter 5). Such estimates are sometimes referred to as "realistic expectations," which are based on statistical information derived from how a large number of people with a specific disease have fared over the short and long term after receiving a particular treatment.

Factors used to determine a person's prognosis may include the size and stage of the tumor, certain features of the tumor observed under the microscope, abnormalities revealed by blood tests, and the tumor's biological properties. People whose tumors have poor prognostic factors may receive more aggressive forms of treatment to improve the outcome. The general health of the person does not usually determine how the cancer will behave, but it can be an important consideration when selecting treatment (see Chapter 4).

Many people with cancer see the staging period as the most difficult period, because it requires numerous trips to the doctor or hospital for tests, and all this time there's still a great deal of uncertainty about treatment and prognosis. It's hard to be patient, but it can be a mistake to rush through things or make a decision based on less than optimum information. It is important to complete all the necessary staging studies before treatment begins, because the information gained helps to "stack the deck" in your favor. In the next chapter we'll look at how decisions about treatment are made using the information gathered during the staging period. With proper staging, the course of treatment can begin with confidence.

Chapter 4

Making Decisions about Treatment: How Success Is Measured

Γhe following are some examples of what a doctor might tell a patient about the chances that a particular treatment will be successful:

— Mr. Johnson, this therapy offers you your only hope.
— Mrs. Olson, if I were in your situation, I would choose this treatment.
— Ms. Jones, your tumor has a 60 percent chance of responding to this treatment.
— Mr. Smith, your chance of successful treatment is 80 percent.

We can deal with the first two statements immediately. What is wrong with the doctor's statement to Mr. Johnson? Although the statement is emotionally persuasive, it is not helpful, because the doctor hasn't told Mr. Johnson what measure of success she is basing her statement on, what side effects of treatment he will experience, or how toxic the treatment is likely to be. Mr. Johnson has no *facts* on which to base a decision about which treatment would be best for him.

What's wrong with the doctor's statement to Mrs. Olson? It's not entirely fair, because her doctor is not in those "shoes," *Mrs. Olson is.* In other words, the doctor and Mrs. Olson have different viewpoints, and the doctor may have failed to take that into account.

The few studies looking at which treatments doctors would choose for themselves indicate that, in general, they would choose the type of treatment they are most familiar with—that is, the type of treatment that is their specialty: the surgeon would choose surgery, the radiation oncologist would choose radiation therapy, and the medical oncologist would choose chemotherapy. Interestingly, the choice of treatment depends not only on the doctor's area of expertise but also on geographic location. A doctor practicing in Europe might well choose a different treatment than a doctor practicing in the United States, and even doctors on the East Coast of the United States and in the Midwest see things differently.

I don't mean that you should not pay attention to your doctor's opinion. I simply want to emphasize that there is no one right answer and that the same information can be interpreted in different ways. In addition, for most cancers, there is more than one appropriate treatment. That is why obtaining a second opinion is as important as having a close working relationship with your primary doctor. In order to make an intelligent decision about your treatment, you must have complete information about the real benefits of various treatments. This chapter describes the information you will need to make an informed decision.

The following general terms are used to define whether a treatment has been successful:

1. the tumor's *response* to treatment
2. the *rate* of response
3. the *duration* of response
4. the patient's chances of *survival*
5. whether the patient's symptoms are reduced and his or her *quality of life* is improved

Keep in mind that the information in this chapter does not apply to a particular type of cancer or to a particular patient. The purpose of the chapter is to help you interpret the information your doctor gives you when discussing your specific disease and to help you make sure that you have all the information you need to make a decision about treatment.

Tumor Response, Response Rate, and Duration

Tumor Response

After the diagnostic and staging tests described in Chapter 3 have been completed, treatment can begin. In the middle and at the end of treatment, the doctor measures the tumor's response to the treatment by repeating some of the earlier tests. When he receives the results of this second round of tests, he has the information he needs to talk with you about how effective your treatment has been. He is likely to use one of the following terms: complete response, partial response, minor response, stable disease, or progressive disease.

Complete response. This response, also referred to as *complete remission,* means that the tumor has disappeared completely. If this is the case, the doctor may say, "You have no evidence of disease" (NED). This doesn't mean that the disease will never return; it means that at this point in time, no disease can be detected.

Partial response. This response, sometimes called *partial remission,* means that the tumor has shrunk to less than half its original size. Precisely how "half" is measured can vary from treatment protocol to treatment protocol. Some protocols define a tumor's size according to its area—by multiplying its length by its width. Other protocols define the size of a tumor according to its volume—by multiplying its length by its width by its thickness. To help standardize response in clinical trials, the National Cancer Institute has developed the Response Evaluation Criteria in Solid Tumors (RECIST criteria) (http://ctep.info.nih.gov/guidelines/recist.html). These criteria are established by panels of experts and are modified periodically as new information and new technologies become available. No matter which measure is used, a partial response means that the tumor has shrunk but is still there. Sometimes, further treatment will turn a partial response into a complete response.

Minor response. Sometimes called a *minor remission,* the term *minor response* means that although the tumor has shrunk, it is still larger than half its original size.

Stable disease. When the term *stable disease* is used, it means that the tumor didn't shrink, but it didn't grow any larger either. *Progressive disease.* This term means that the tumor has become at least 25 percent larger than it was before treatment.

If a patient has more than one tumor, the overall response is determined by the tumor with the worst response. For example, if a patient has three tumors and, after treatment, one has disappeared, the second has shrunk to less than half its original size, and the third has become at least 25 percent larger than it was before treatment, the disease is still called progressive, although two tumors responded well to treatment.

Response Rate

The term *response rate* refers to the *likelihood* that a tumor will either shrink or disappear after a specific treatment. The categories of response described in the previous section are used to define how an individual patient's tumor has responded to treatment. However, most studies determine how large groups of patients respond to a particular treatment; thus, doctors speak of the "rate" of a particular response to the treatment in a large group of patients.

For example, let's say that in a group of 100 patients, the rate of complete response (or complete remission) is 30 percent. In other words, the tumors of 30 patients disappeared as the result of treatment. The remaining 70 patients had either a partial or a minor response, stable disease, or progressive disease. In another group of 100 patients, the tumors of 25 patients have disappeared completely, and the tumors of another 35 patients have shrunk to less than half their original size. In this group of patients, the overall response rate to treatment is 60 percent—25 percent complete response and 35 percent partial response. The remaining 40 patients had a minor response, stable disease, or progressive disease.

When you and your doctor discuss your treatment options, she might describe your likelihood of responding to a particular treatment in the terms that Ms. Jones' doctor used: "You have a 60 percent chance of responding to this treatment." In this case, the doctor is probably telling you that the chance your tumor will *either disappear or be reduced by half* is 60 percent. For most treatments, these two clinical response categories are important, because patients who respond completely or partially to a treatment will do best in the long run.

The responses of the patients who do not achieve a complete or partial remission also may indicate success. Some large tumors may shrink a little and remain stable indefinitely because the part of the tumor that disappeared may be replaced by massive scar tissue resulting from the tumor and the healing process. This could happen with Hodgkin's disease, when a mass might shrink a little and then stay that way for many years because it is now just scar tissue; over time it may shrink even more. In other words, for all practical purposes, Bob has been "cured," because no cancer cells are present. More often, however, patients who don't have a complete response usually require more treatment.

Now let's examine Mr. Smith's doctor's statement—"Your chance of successful treatment is 80 percent." The doctor has not told Mr. Smith what she is using to *measure* success. She *might* mean that there is an 80 percent chance that the surgeon will be able to remove all of Mr. Smith's tumor. On the other hand, she might mean that the response rate of Mr. Smith's type of tumor to chemotherapy or radiotherapy is 80 percent. To fully understand what the doctor means, Mr. Smith should ask the doctor for a complete explanation of the measure of success that she is using.

Duration of Response

In addition to knowing your chances of having a complete response to a particular treatment, you need to know how long the remission is likely to last—in other words, its duration. Some remissions are permanent, meaning that the disease has been cured, whereas others may last only a few months. The reason that complete remissions are so important is that they are usually the only ones that will last a long time or be permanent. Although partial remissions and stable disease are usually not permanent, they, too, can be important because they add time and comfort to a patient's life.

Survival

Survival refers to how long a patient may live and the likelihood that the disease will return (recur) at some point. Survival is defined in two important ways: *overall survival* and *disease-free survival*. Both types of survival are based on mathematical curves generated by experts in statistics. Survival curves are, in a sense, estimates of outcome. As the duration of patient follow-up increases, so does the accuracy of the estimate. The average duration of follow-up is called the *median follow-up*. Estimates too far beyond the median follow-up are not too accurate. For example, if there is a median follow-up of 4 years, the estimate of survival at 7 years would not be very accurate and may change as the duration of follow-up increases. Examples of overall and disease-free survival curves are shown in figure 4.1. Such curves are produced to show the outcomes of different treatments for the same type of cancer, making it easy to compare the different treatments.

Note that at the bottom of figure 4.1 (the *x* axis, "Years from start of treatment") the number of years begins at 0 and ends at 10; 0 represents the beginning of treatment. All survival curves begin at Time 0. Time 0 is when a patient starts treatment; it is not a date on the calendar. The time on the *x* axis is, then, the time from the start of treatment. On the left-hand side of the graph—the *y* axis, "Percentage (%)"—the percentages begin at 0 and end at 100. Assuming that 100 patients have started treatment is the easiest way to present this discussion.

Overall Survival

The overall survival curve in figure 4.1 tells us the percentage of patients who are likely to be alive at different time points. Because all the patients were alive when treatment began (Time 0), the curve begins at 100 percent. Four years after Time 0, as you can see, 80 percent of the patients (80 out of 100) are likely to be alive. The curve also indicates that 10 years after treatment began, approximately two-thirds (65%) of the 100 patients are likely to be alive. Because no one lives forever, the overall survival percentages, obviously, will continue to fall over time.

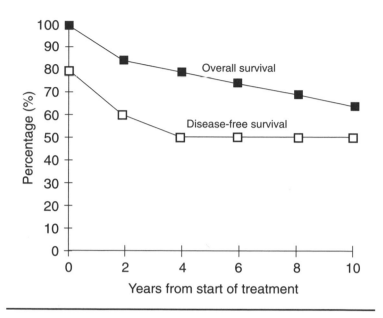

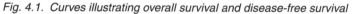

Fig. 4.1. Curves illustrating overall survival and disease-free survival

The survival curves are calculated from large groups of people with the same disease. They are used to compare different treatments and can be useful in estimating the outcome for an individual.

An overall survival curve does *not* indicate whether a remission is permanent or whether the disease has recurred. In addition, you need to keep in mind that when statisticians calculate overall survival curves, they include deaths from all causes—for example, heart attacks and accidents as well as cancer. Deaths that are unrelated to cancer are sometimes called *intercurrent deaths*.

Disease-Free Survival

Disease-free survival (freedom from progression of the tumor) is a measure of how many patients are alive and have no evidence of cancer at some point after treatment. Disease-free survival is usually the best measure of successful treatment and is often the most useful of all the survival curves.

The lower curve in figure 4.1 indicates the percentages of patients who have had no evidence of disease at different time points since Time 0. Because only 80 of the 100 patients were in complete remission when their treatment ended, this curve begins at 80 percent rather than 100 percent; the cancer never disappeared in the other 20 percent. The curve indicates that at 2 years, 60 percent of the patients remain free of cancer and will have not experienced a recurrence. The other 40 percent either did not have a complete remission to begin with (the first 20 percent who never appeared on the figure), or, if they did have a complete remission, the disease has recurred.

Note that this curve falls to 50 percent at 4 years. Also note that the curve flattens out after 4 years because the disease has not recurred in the remaining patients, and the remission is permanent. This flattening may be called a *plateau*.

On the basis of the curve for disease-free survival, one could say that 50 percent of the patients were cured by their initial treatment. In reality, however, the number of patients who are doing well may be even higher, because some patients whose disease recurred may go into remission again with additional treatment.

Again, let's examine the statement that the doctor made to Mr. Smith: "Your chance of successful treatment is 80 percent." She might be referring to a point on either curve. If she is referring to either the overall survival curve or the disease-free curve, she should tell Mr. Smith which curve and point in time she is referring to. For example, "Mr. Smith, your chance of disease-free survival at 4 years is 50 percent" would be useful information. Again, if Mr. Smith is uncertain about what measure of success the doctor is using, he should ask for more information.

Other Information Provided by the Two Curves

Different types of cancers have different rates of relapse. For some rapidly growing tumors such as aggressive lymphomas, the disease-free survival curve will reach a plateau after just a few years, whereas for slowly growing tumors, such as low-grade lymphomas, prostate cancer, or breast cancer, the rate of relapse may be constant over many years. For both rapid- and slow-growing tumors, survival may be excellent, but because a survival curve includes all causes of mortality, it will fall continuously over time. Generally speaking, however, most patients who relapse will do so in the years immediately after treatment ends rather than later. Consequently, the doctor is likely to tell you the percentages at 5 years after treatment. To fully understand the percentage, it is important to know both the type of survival and the time elapsed.

When you are in the process of discussing and selecting your treatment, your doctor may give you the percentages of overall and disease-free survival for two different types of treatment, such as surgery and radiation therapy. He should give you the rates of complete remission for each treatment, the rates of overall and disease-free survival for each treatment, and the side effects of each one.

An *extremely important point* to keep in mind is that a difference between the two treatments of a few percentage points, or a difference of even 10 percent or more, does not necessarily mean that one treatment is better than the other. This is especially true if the curves for each treatment were constructed from the results obtained from two different research studies or from two very different periods of time.

The percentages in these curves are not precise. If the same treatment is studied at two different treatment centers, the percentages may be slightly different. Some curves may represent an *average* of the results obtained from a *number* of studies. An average percentage may represent a range: for example, if the average response rate is 50 percent, the actual percentages obtained in different studies may have ranged from 40 percent to 60 percent. (In statistics, an average number or percentage is called the *mean,* and the range is expressed as the *standard deviation.*)

Another factor that may affect the percentages is the health of the patients who participated in different studies. For example, if younger, healthier patients receive surgery and older, sicker patients receive radiation therapy, the surgery may appear to be more successful than radiation therapy although the two treatments are actually equally successful because the first group of patients was healthier to begin with. Let's assume that we are comparing the results of treatment for bladder cancer with radiation and surgery. When the doctor considers which patients should undergo a major surgical procedure, he usually recommends it for the healthiest patients; radiation therapy is recommended for patients who are less healthy. That makes sense, because patients whose general health is poor may not do well under the stress of anesthesia and surgery. There are performance status scales that can describe the activity level of a patient. Two scales commonly used are the ECOG and the Karnofsky status scale; these are included in Appendix C.

Meaningful comparisons can be made between two different treatments only if the doctor and the patient realize that the doctors who conducted different studies exercised some bias when deciding which patients should receive which treatment. This is one reason that clinical trials are so important: They can take into account the general health of the patients who participate and consequently provide a more accurate measure of the success and side effects of the different treatments.

Other Methods of Assessing the Success of Treatment

Quality of Life

One important goal of cancer treatment is to achieve the best quality of life possible for the patient, even for the patient who cannot be cured. Toxicity scoring systems are used to assess the acute and long-term toxicity of treatment, discussed in the next chapter. The Common Terminology Criteria for Adverse Events (CTCAE), developed by the NCI with expert panels, is used for NCI and other clinical trials groups (http://ctep.cancer. gov/forms/CTCAEv3.pdf).

Researchers in psychosocial oncology—a relatively new field devoted to the psychological and social ramifications of cancer and its treatments—have developed questionnaires that measure how the patient feels, how much time he or she spends in normal activities, and how he or she interacts with other people, including family members. Quality-of-life assessment is an important part of clinical research, because it helps determine how much benefit patients actually derive from their treatment. If two treatments are approximately equal in their ability to cure the cancer but one leaves the person less able to live a normal life, then the choice of treatment will depend both on its potential for success and on how functional the person will be for the rest of his or her life. Appendix B gives more details about the concept of quality-adjusted life years, which is an attempt to add an assessment of quality of life to quantity.

Competing-Risk Analysis

Competing-risk analysis is used to determine which treatment is most appropriate for a specific patient. Before evaluating an individual patient's treatment options, the doctor must consider the following questions:

— When will the patient's cancer progress and what problems is it likely to cause?
— Will the patient develop complications as a result of a particular treatment?
— Will the patient have serious problems caused by other medical problems that are unrelated to the cancer (severe heart disease, for example)?

To make the best decision, the doctor relies on information such as the following:

1. the life span of the average person in the population;
2. the risk that the patient's cancer will recur at some point after treatment and the pattern of its progression (the parts of the body to which it is likely to spread, the symptoms it is likely to cause, the time course of its progression without treatment, and the success rate of treatment when the cancer recurs or progresses);
3. the availability of effective second-line or salvage treatment should the cancer recur after the initial treatment;
4. the risk that the patient will develop acute complications

during therapy and will develop late complications as a result of treatment; and

5. any non–cancer-related diseases the patient may have—for information about a specific patient with heart disease, for example, the doctor would consult the patient's heart specialist.

In other words, two patients with the same cancer diagnosis and stage of disease might receive different treatments on the basis of the doctor's assessment of competing risks.

Meta Analysis

A statistical tool called a *meta analysis* is used to combine mathematically the results of a group of studies of the treatment of a specific disease to see if there is an improvement for patients undergoing that particular treatment. For studies to be statistically significant, there must be enough patients to detect a difference between one treatment and another. If one treatment is much better, a small study will do; however, for most clinical trials the difference is usually modest, perhaps a 5 to 10 percent improvement. Identifying a statistically significant difference between treatments may require many hundreds or even thousands of patients.

The meta analysis allows a statistician to combine the results for a group of studies—although each of the studies is too small to prove a difference, the composite may do so. Showing a statistically significant difference is important because one treatment may look better than another by chance alone. In essence, there is security in numbers by combining studies. An example of the benefit of the meta analysis is in the use of adjuvant therapy for women with breast cancer. Many studies showed a small improvement, but it took a meta analysis of many thousands of patients to demonstrate that the small difference was indeed "real." This positive result helped patients and physicians decide what to do and also helped those who finance health care to know that the money for such adjuvant treatment is justified with a real potential benefit. There are potential downsides to a meta analysis, in that the composition of the individual trials may not be comparable so that overall result is not truly meaningful. Thus, these studies are helpful but must be interpreted with care.

Other Types of Survival Curves

Although the curves illustrated in figure 4.1 are used most often, other types of survival curves, such as those described below, can also be used to determine the success of treatment.

Cause-specific survival. Cause-specific survival, also called *determinate survival,* is a measure of how many people have died from their cancer or its treatment. The curve is similar to an overall survival curve except that it only counts deaths related to cancer; it does not count deaths from other causes. This measure is not always accurate, because it is not always possible to determine whether a patient died from cancer or its treatment or from other causes.

Cause-specific survival curves will always look better than overall survival curves. Here's why: Let's assume that a group of older patients has been treated for a certain type of cancer. Five years after treatment began (Time 0), only 60 percent of the patients are alive: that is, 60 out of 100 are still living, and 40 have died. However, among the 40 patients who died, 15 died from heart attacks and only 25 patients died from cancer or its treatment. This means that 5 years after Time 0, the cause-specific survival is 75 percent, whereas the overall survival would be 60 percent. A cause-specific survival curve will yield a higher percentage than an overall survival curve will.

Relapse-free survival. Relapse-free survival curves, also called freedom-from-relapse curves, are usually used to describe the frequency of recurrence among patients who had achieved a complete remission. Because these curves only include patients who originally achieved a complete remission, the results will look better than those in disease-free survival curves, which include patients who achieved a complete remission, patients whose cancer did not disappear, and patients who achieved a complete remission but experienced a recurrence.

Again, let's assume that in a group of 100 patients who received a certain treatment, 80 percent achieved a complete remission. Among those 80 patients, 20 have recurrent disease. Therefore, of the 100 original patients, 60 percent are doing well. The disease-free survival curve would include all 100 patients in the calculations: the 60 patients who remain in remission, the 20 whose disease recurred after remission, and the 20 who did not achieve a complete remission in the first place. Thus, the rate of disease-free survival is 60 percent. Because the relapse-free survival curve includes only 80 patients (only those who had a complete remission), 20 of whom have relapsed, the rate of relapse-free survival is 75 percent: that is, 60 of the 80 patients (or three-fourths) with a complete remission have not relapsed. Therefore, the relapse-free survival curve has a higher percentage of success than a disease-free survival curve does.

Failure-free survival. Failure-free survival curves include all causes of an unfavorable outcome. Included among the "failures" are patients who never achieved a complete remission; those who achieved a complete remission, then relapsed; and those who died from any cause, cancer related or non–cancer related. Because the curve will fall if any bad event occurs, failure-free survival will have the lowest percentage of successful outcomes of any of the curves described.

In this chapter I have described the basic concepts on which rates of remission are based, and I have explained survival curves. All the information in this chapter and the next one will be extremely helpful when you discuss treatment options with your doctors and your family. The next chapter describes how a patient can make certain that he or she has the appropriate information for weighing the potential risks of treatment against the potential benefits.

Chapter 5

Weighing the Long-Term Risks and Benefits of Treatment

Most cancer patients do not develop adverse effects later in life as a result of their treatment, but some patients do eventually experience damage to an organ such as the heart or the lung, and some patients develop a treatment-related secondary cancer. For this reason, when oncologists design a treatment regimen for individual patients, they take into account the risk of late effects associated with the treatment. The late effects are included in the CTCAE (described in Chapter 4). Because it often takes years for the late effects of treatment to develop, most studies of late effects have involved adults who survived leukemia in childhood or Hodgkin's disease in young adulthood. The cure rate for both diseases is extremely high, and patients survive for many decades after treatment.

Oncologists weigh the risks associated with different treatments against the benefits of those treatments by estimating the *risk-benefit ratio.* When determining a person's risk of developing a *late effect of treatment,* oncologists rely on one of two methods of calculating estimates of risk: *relative risk* and *actuarial risk.* Because these methods are complicated, doctors usually don't discuss them in any detail with patients. But patients need to understand these methods in order to make sense of the advice doctors give when comparing treatment outcomes and prognosis. In this chapter I explain how oncologists arrive at estimates of risk and how they compare those risks with the benefits of treatment. A discussion of risk-benefit ratios comes first, followed by a more detailed discussion of how the numbers and percentages are arrived at. The risk of developing a secondary cancer is used as an example of a late toxicity. (This chapter both expands on material that was introduced in Chapter 4 and introduces new concepts.)

Risk-Benefit Ratio

An essential part of making a decision about which treatment is best for you is an assessment of what is called the *risk-benefit ratio;* this applies to any decision one makes in life. For example, what are the risks versus benefits of changing your job, investing in Stock X versus Stock Y, or taking a train rather than a plane? What is considered to be a reasonable risk of selecting a given treatment depends on what benefits the treatment will provide.

Let's look at how the risks and benefits of a particular treatment are weighed.

— What if there is a 50 percent chance that the treatment will be successful and the chances of developing late toxicity are 0? Anyone would choose that treatment.

— What if there is a 75 percent chance that the treatment will be successful and the risk of serious toxicity is only 5 percent? Almost everyone would choose that treatment.

— What if there is a 30 percent chance that the treatment will be successful and the risk that the eventual toxicity will be fatal is 25 percent? This treatment would seem to be a reasonable choice if the risk of dying from the cancer within 6 months is extremely high.

— What if the chance that the treatment will be successful is only 5 percent and there is a 20 percent chance that it will be fatal? Few people would see this as an attractive choice.

— What if there is no chance that the treatment will be curative but it will buy the person some time? People faced with a choice like this must decide on the basis of their own personal situation, the risks they are willing to accept, and whether the side effects of the treatment seem reasonable.

Deciding which treatment option is best for you is a personal choice. To help you make the best decision, your doctor will provide you with the most accurate estimates possible concerning the risks and benefits of each treatment option available to you. By writing down this information on your Patient's Checklist and studying the information carefully, you and your family will be able to decide which treatment option is most worthwhile.

Risk of Late Complications
Relative Risk

In any group of people, there is a risk that some of them will develop cancer during their lifetime. This risk is called the *expected number* of cancers. When the number of cured cancer patients who develop secondary cancers later in life is calculated, the result is the *observed number* of cancers.

To calculate the relative risk, the number of observed cases is divided by the number of expected cases:

$$\text{Relative risk} = \frac{\text{Observed cases}}{\text{Expected cases}}$$

Statistical methods are then applied to see whether more former patients than expected developed secondary cancers some years after their first cancer was cured. For example, let's say a group of 1,000 adults were cured of Hodgkin's disease when they were young adults. Fifteen years later, we find that 36 of these former patients have developed leukemia, but we expected only 4 people in 1,000 who have never had Hodgkin's disease to develop this leukemia. Therefore, to determine the relative risk that former Hodgkin's patients will develop leukemia later in life, we would divide 36 by 4, which is 9. In other words, there are 9 times more cases of leukemia than we would have expected.

Although the relative risk of 9 seems high, only 36 (about 3.5%) of the 1,000 patients developed this complication, whereas 964 did not, and 4 of the 1,000 patients would have developed leukemia whether they had had Hodgkin's disease or not. Therefore, only 32 (about 3%) of 1,000 patients developed leukemia because of their earlier Hodgkin's disease or its treatment.

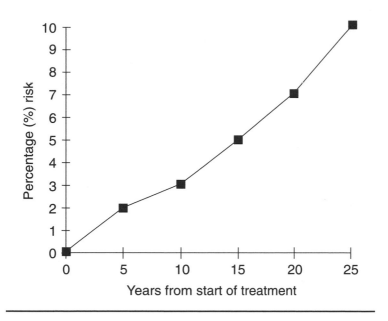

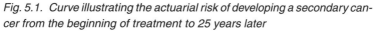

Fig. 5.1. Curve illustrating the actuarial risk of developing a secondary cancer from the beginning of treatment to 25 years later

As with all actuarial curves, this is a statistical estimate. This curve includes cancers that occurred as the result of the disease and its treatment and cancers that would have occurred naturally.

Actuarial Risk

Using the actuarial risk, the second method of defining the risk of developing a secondary cancer, makes it easier to understand what the risk means to an individual patient. Figure 5.1 is a curve for the actuarial risk of developing a secondary cancer. It is similar in concept to the curves discussed in Chapter 4. The major difference is that the curves for actuarial risk of complications go up, not down like survival curves.

For example, when William, a young man with Hodgkin's disease, begins receiving treatment (Time 0), no secondary tumors have occurred. Therefore, his actuarial risk of developing a secondary cancer at Time 0 is 0 percent. Ten years later, however, his actuarial risk is 3 percent, which means that of 100 Hodgkin's patients who are alive 10 years after treatment, William may be one of three who have developed a secondary tumor—a number that continues to rise over time. Thus, as the curve indicates, at 20 years after Time 0, William's actuarial risk of developing a secondary cancer increases to 7 percent.

Actuarial curves indicate the total number of former patients who eventually developed a secondary cancer. It is important to realize, however, that many of these secondary cancers can be cured and that you must be cured of your first cancer to be at risk for late complications. Another important consideration is that because cancer becomes more common as we get older, some of the risk is from the Hodgkin's disease and its treatment, and some is simply the risk from life itself. Using the knowledge we have about late complications, doctors have now modified chemotherapy and radiation therapy regimens to reduce the risk of late toxicity. Additional screening is done for patients who are at increased risk.

Prognosis

In simple terms, a *prognosis* is a statistical estimate of the chance that a patient will be alive at a certain point in time after treatment; it is based on average numbers for a large group of patients. Thus, the answer to the famous question "How long do I have, Doc?" can only ever be an *average*—and the nature of averages means that some people do better and some people do worse than the average. Understanding the survival curves described in Chapter 4 is helpful here, and especially during the discussion of the factors that influence who gets which treatment. Estimates of prognosis are not particularly accurate, for the following reasons:

— Not all people who are diagnosed with cancer are in the same age group.
— Different people's tumors have different characteristics.
— People have different abilities to undergo certain treatments.

— Different people differ with regard to a variety of other factors.

Furthermore, because treatments improve over time, the best information available about prognosis may not necessarily apply to today's treatments. For example, the major breakthrough of Gleevec® for chronic myelogenous leukemia led to a dramatic improvement in outcome. Thus, it is impossible to predict a specific individual's prognosis with complete accuracy.

The type of information that doctors frequently use when discussing a prognosis with a patient is the chance that the patient will be alive or free of disease at a certain point in time, often at 5 years. For example, a 5-year survival of 70 percent means that at 5 years, 70 out of 100 patients are likely to be alive. But remember that some of the 30 percent will have died from noncancer causes. The other common estimate is the *median survival*—the point at which half the patients will still be alive. For example, if the median survival time is 4 years, half of the patients will still be alive at that point. (Median survival is discussed in more detail below.)

For a variety of legitimate reasons, many patients only want to know what their prognosis is in general terms, not in specific percentages. Other patients ask the doctor to make a specific prognosis, so they can use this information to help them in planning their future. Although such an estimate may be useful in planning, it is in no way a guarantee.

Because (for the reasons stated above) a precise prognosis cannot be determined, your doctor is not being evasive when he gives you a range of numbers or what amounts to his best "guesstimate." It is important to recognize that statistics apply to *groups* of patients, not to any one person. Either a specific treatment will be effective for a specific patient or will not. For many cancers, there are secondary treatments available if the first treatment is unsuccessful. Therefore, although percentages are helpful in understanding the general prognosis and in selecting the treatment, it is impossible to predict the course for any individual patient with certainty.

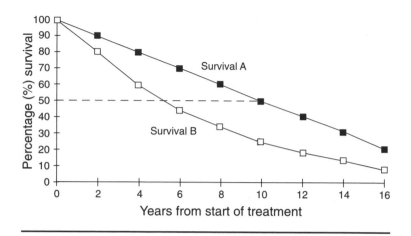

Fig. 5.2. Curves illustrating median survival times for two groups of people with the same type of cancer

The patients with Stage A disease have localized tumors with no involvement of lymph nodes. Those with Stage B have localized tumors of the same size as the other group, but a few lymph nodes are involved. The median survival time is the time at which the curves cross 50 percent survival.

Estimates Concerning Prognosis

Figure 5.2 contains two hypothetical overall survival curves for two groups of patients with different stages of the same type of cancer—Stage A or Stage B. For this discussion, let's assume that the patients with Stage A disease have a localized tumor and the lymph nodes in the region are not involved. The patients with Stage B disease have localized tumors that are the same size as the tumors in Stage A patients, but in Stage B disease a few lymph nodes in the region are involved. In other words, the disease of the Stage B group is slightly more advanced. Let's also assume that the patients in both groups receive the best treatment available.

When looking at the overall survival curves, keep in mind that they include deaths from all causes. The time when the curve falls to 50 percent (when half the patients have died and half are still alive) is called the *median survival time* (indicated by the broken line drawn across the graph at 50 percent). Looking at the upper curve, we see that 75 percent of the patients with Stage A disease are alive at 5 years, 50 percent are alive at 10 years, and 25 percent are alive at 15 years. The median survival time for the patients in this group is 10 years. The lower curve shows that the median survival time for patients with Stage B disease is 5 years (the point where the broken line crosses the curve). In both curves, however, some patients are still alive at 16 years.

So, what should your doctor say when you ask her about your prognosis? All she can do is give you a projection based on these survival curves. If you had Stage A disease, she could say, "You have 10 years," which is the median survival time; however, you might live less than 10 years or longer than 10 years. If you had Stage B disease and asked your doctor for a prognosis, she could point out that although the median survival time is 5 years, 50 percent of patients with Stage B disease live longer than that.

Methods of Comparing Different Treatment Outcomes

Survival curves can also be used to compare the benefits of two different treatments. The hypothetical disease-free survival curves shown in figure 5.3 compare Treatment P and Treatment Q for patients with the same stage of disease. The difference between the two curves can be compared in two ways: by the *vertical difference method* or by the *horizontal difference method*.

Vertical difference method. The vertical difference is the most commonly used method of comparing treatment outcomes. The curves are compared at a specific time, and the difference in the two percentages at that time is compared. For example, at 5 years, 60 percent of the patients who received Treatment P have not relapsed, whereas 50 percent of the patients who received Treatment Q have not relapsed. Thus, the difference between the two treatment outcomes 5 years after Time 0 is 10 percent. Note that 8 years after the treatments began, 32 percent of the patients who received Treatment P have not relapsed, whereas 28 percent of the patients who received Treatment Q have not relapsed. Thus, 8 years after Time 0, there is a small difference of only 4 percent.

Horizontal difference method. With this method, the horizontal difference between the curves is used; this difference is the

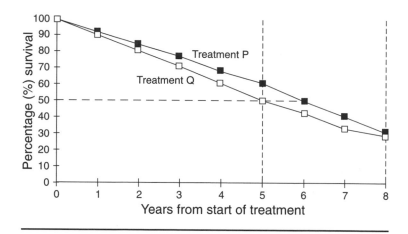

Fig. 5.3. Curves illustrating hypothetical disease-free survival for two groups of patients who received different treatments

One group received Treatment P and the other Treatment Q. The curves can be compared two ways. In vertical comparison, the difference in percentage disease-free survival can be compared at various points in time, as illustrated at 5 and 8 years. In horizontal comparison, the number of years required to reach the median survival is compared. Illustrated with the horizontal broken line is the comparison of median (50%) survival.

time when each curve reaches a certain percentage of survival. In figure 5.3, the horizontal broken line indicates the time when both curves reach the median disease-free survival of 50 percent. Note that the patients who received Treatment Q reached the 50 percent mark at 5 years, whereas the patients who received Treatment P reached the 50 percent mark at 6 years, a difference of 1 year. Any other relationships between times and percentages can be compared in the same way. Note that at 8 years the percentages of patients in the two groups who have not relapsed are almost identical. Statisticians can compare two survival curves by measuring the hazard ratio. Each curve in figure 5.3 falls at a certain rate, called the *hazard rate*. The ratio of hazard rates is the hazard ratio. Applying statistical analysis to the hazard ratio, which depends on the number of patients represented by each of the curves, allows the statistician to determine whether the difference is "statistically significant." Clinical trials are designed so that there are enough people studied to draw a meaningful conclusion.

As this example shows, the difference between the treatments can vary, depending on whether vertical or horizontal differences are used for comparison or when, in time, the comparison is made. There is no "right" time to look at the curves and see which treatment is better. In the case of diseases with survival statistics that are not good for many patients (indicated by a rapid fall between Time 0 and 5 years for both treatments), a more important time point may be near the end of the survival curves, where the percentages of survival between the treatments may be farther apart.

In some situations, an extremely aggressive treatment may be available which carries with it the possibility not only of a cure but also of a high risk of death. As a result, the survival statistics for that treatment may be lower than those for a milder treatment in the early years after Time 0, but they may be higher than the statistics for the milder treatment over the long term. In fact, the two survival curves may actually cross in the long run.

In other situations, the results of different treatments may be similar, but one treatment produces a better quality of life than the other treatment does. Thus, some patients may choose to "give up a few percentage points" at 5 to 10 years to achieve a better quality of life. For example, some patients with head and neck, bladder, or rectal cancer may choose to preserve their organs rather than have them surgically removed, even though this decision *may* shorten their lives to some minor extent.

Reporting of Treatment Benefits

This section will explain how differently the results of a clinical trial can be described in news reports or in medical journals. The two disease-free survival curves in figure 5.3 can be used to illustrate the problem.

At 5 years, the disease-free survival for Treatment P is 60 percent, whereas it is 50 percent for Treatment Q. Thus, the "absolute difference" between the two percentages is 10 percent, so this number could be reported. However, the "percentage reduction" in the number of patients who relapsed after Treatment P is better by 20 percent than it is for Treatment Q in the following way: 50 percent of the patients who received Treatment Q have relapsed at 5 years, 40 percent of the patients who received Treatment P have relapsed. So, the benefit of Treatment P versus Treatment Q is the difference of 10 percent divided by the percentage of relapses after Treatment Q, which is 50 percent: 10 percent divided by 50 percent = 20 percent. In other words, 10 of the 50 patients who relapsed after Treatment Q would not have relapsed if they had received Treatment P. Although only 10 percent of the patients who received Treatment P are doing better than are those who received Treatment Q, the result can legitimately be reported as a 20 percent "reduction in relapse" for Treatment P.

What if two different treatments are highly successful? What if the patients who received Treatment X have a 5-year rate of relapse-free survival of 97 percent and those who received Treatment Y have a 5-year rate of relapse-free survival of 91 percent? The absolute difference in relapse-free survival at 5 years is 6 percent. However, 3 percent of the patients experience a relapse with Treatment X and 9 percent experience a relapse with Treatment Y. Of the 9 patients who relapsed with Treatment Y, 6 would not have relapsed if they had received Treatment X. Therefore, the percentage reduction in relapse for Treatment X compared with Treatment Y is 9 percent minus 3 percent = 6 percent, and 6 percent divided by 9 percent = 67 percent. Thus, a treatment that appears to benefit only 6 out of 100 patients can be reported as a 67 percent reduction in the risk of relapse with Treatment X compared with Treatment Y.

As you can see, when percentage benefits are presented, especially in news reports, the reader or listener must be aware of the different ways in which the same results can be stated. A basic understanding of survival curves will make it easy to understand the real benefits of one treatment compared with another.

Outcomes Analysis

As media reports on health care reform clearly show, the issues involved in the process of health care reform are extremely complex. Outcomes analysis is one of these issues. As health care providers try to determine which treatments are "appropriate" or "best" for a specific illness, outcomes analysis, which involves estimating the costs and benefits of different treatments, has come to be an important factor in their decisions. When deciding which treatments will be used by an entire country, an insurance plan, or an individual, such estimates are crucially important.

Because cancer is a common disease and screening, prevention, treatment, and research can be expensive, patients and their families are often confronted with cost-effectiveness issues. These issues can be especially stressful when they involve new and expensive therapies and technologies. The process used to consider the available treatment options is called *decision analysis*. Various mathematical models can be used. Because the results of decision analyses usually apply to a large population of patients, the numbers represent averages and will not apply to a specific patient. (The terms and concepts used in decision analysis are discussed in Appendix B.)

Responsible development of new treatments and technologies requires rigorous research standards and careful attention to treatment outcomes, both in years of life gained and in quality of life. New treatments and technologies are generally expensive, and for the benefits of patients and society, vigorous efforts must be made to contain their costs. These efforts include avoiding the impulse to apply new treatments before they have been carefully evaluated. That is why it is so helpful for eligible patients to participate in clinical trials and for the results of clinical trials to be reported in an appropriate and timely manner.

Although the investigator's and the patients' enthusiasm for a new treatment is laudable, exaggerating the results of the treatment or publicizing them prematurely or incompletely may lead to unjustifiable hope as well as to unjustifiable expense on the patient's part. Furthermore, exaggeration or premature publication may lead to an improper allocation of resources—either spending too much on a treatment that is not particularly beneficial or losing the opportunity to examine the benefits and costs of a new treatment or technological advance carefully before it is introduced into routine practice.

In this chapter I have discussed the various ways in which the risks of treatment can be compared with the benefits of treatment. In the next chapter I turn to a discussion of the three standard methods of treating cancer and an explanation of how these treatments can be used alone, in combination, or in sequence to provide the best treatment outcome for the person with cancer. In Chapter 7 I discuss the emerging molecular-targeted treatments.

Chapter 6

Conventional Treatments: An Overview

This chapter focuses primarily on the three standard methods of treating cancer: surgery, chemotherapy, and radiation therapy. Brief descriptions of newer treatment modalities, such as bone marrow transplantation and hormonal therapies, are also included here. Molecular-targeted treatment is discussed in Chapter 7, while clinical trials testing new treatments are described in Chapter 8.

Your doctors will provide you with detailed information about your treatment options. Other sources of information are also available, including medical textbooks as well as books and articles written for the general public, on-line chat groups, and educational Web sites (for a list of some recommended readings, see the bibliography). Organizations such as the National Cancer Institute, the American Cancer Society, and the National Comprehensive Cancer Network provide useful printed materials, and information is available from computer services such as the PDQ system listed in Chapter 1.

Treatment Modalities and Informed Consent

When a person's cancer is treated using only one treatment modality, this is called *monotherapy* or *single-modality therapy*. When more than one treatment modality is used, the term is *combination therapy* or *multimodality therapy*. Combination therapies can be administered at the same time (simultaneously), one after the other (sequentially), or in alternating cycles. When more than one treatment is administered simultaneously, the specialists involved must coordinate and schedule the treatments carefully. In one common sequential treatment, either surgery or radiation therapy is used first, to remove or shrink the tumor mass. This is followed by chemotherapy to treat any cells that may have metastasized.

Most cancer treatments are designed to cure the disease either by removing the tumor or by killing all the cancer cells. Sometimes, however, cure is impossible. The goal of treatment in these cases is to reduce the patients' symptoms, improve their quality of life, and prolong their lives. This kind of treatment is called *palliative care.*

Because different people with the same diagnosis and stage of disease will differ in characteristics such as age or general health, an oncologist must consider the competing risks described in Chapter 5 when determining which treatment is best for each individual. In addition, the oncologist must consider three additional concerns: whether the cancer is confined to the primary (local) tumor, whether other nearby (regional) tissues are involved, and whether cancer cells may have metastasized to distant sites.

Whatever type of treatment you receive, you will be given an *informed consent form* to read—carefully—and sign. In addition to giving the doctor and the treating institution permission to provide the treatment, this form describes the treatment and all of its likely or possible side effects, which can include physical symptoms (such as nausea), abnormal blood tests (low blood counts), and abnormal results of imaging tests (so that, for example, future x-rays may show an abnormality where a tumor has been treated with radiation). Although the extensive list of side effects in the informed consent form is necessary, in part for legal reasons, it can be frightening. However, most people experience only a few of the side effects described in the form. Many forms, in fact, subdivide side effects into those that are acute and late and those that are common, uncommon, rare, and extremely rare.

Acute side effects occur during treatment and usually disappear a few days or weeks after treatment ends. Their severity is usually graded on a scale of 1 to 4 or 5. Grade 1 side effects are usually mild and may be barely noticeable. People who experience Grade 2 or 3 side effects may need a drug such as an antibiotic to cure an infection, an antiemetic to relieve nausea, or a drug to control pain (and methods of controlling pain have been greatly improved). Many people who develop Grade 4 or 5 side effects must be hospitalized —their symptoms may be life-threatening. In some cases, the cancer treatment may need to be changed because of the side effects.

Finally, as described in Chapter 1, it is very important for you to make regular follow-up visits to your oncologists as well as to your primary care doctor after your treatment has been completed. All people who have had cancer need to be checked for a recurrence of their disease and any late effects that may develop. These visits become less frequent as time passes.

Surgery

Most people are familiar with the purpose of surgical procedures. The goal of cancer surgery is to remove the tumor while maintaining the affected organ's ability to function, if possible. The routine for cancer surgery is similar to the routine involved in any surgical procedure: you may need to have routine diagnostic tests (blood tests and x-rays) before surgery, you will need to stop food and fluids for a specified period before surgery, and so on. Your doctor will tell you what to expect and will probably give you a printed sheet with presurgical instructions for the patient.

To make appropriate plans at home and at work, ask your surgeon these questions:

— How long will I be in the hospital?
— Will I lose much blood?
— Will I need radiation therapy or chemotherapy after the operation?
— Am I likely to have permanent physical problems because of the surgery?
— How long will my recovery (or rehabilitation) take?

If your surgery will involve loss of blood and you are likely to need a transfusion during the procedure, you may want to donate your own blood (called *autologous blood banking*) a few weeks before the surgery.

Surgery is sometimes performed to *debulk* a tumor—to remove most, but not all, of the tumor. Although debulking may prolong a person's life, it may produce side effects that have a negative effect on the person's quality of life without affecting the outcome of the disease. Therefore, the decision to undergo this type of surgery is a difficult one.

In cancer treatment, surgical procedures are also used to restore function to an organ that has been partially removed or to insert an implant (*prosthesis*) that takes the place of an organ that has been completely removed. These types of surgeries are called *reconstructive surgery.*

Innovative surgical techniques now being used require a less extensive surgical procedure. This includes sentinel node biopsy to help stage tumors such as breast cancer and melanoma. This biopsy involves injecting a colored dye or radioactive tracer near the tumor and removal of the nodes to which the dye or tracer tracks. *Minimally invasive surgery* can also be performed for a number of diseases in the abdomen (through a procedure called *laparoscopy*) and chest (*thoracoscopy*) using video-assisted techniques. Additionally, partial organ removal may be possible in cancers such as kidney or pancreas cancer, thereby making life easier for the patient than having the entire organ removed.

Radiation therapy or chemotherapy (or both) is often used in combination with limited surgery so that part of an organ can be preserved. One common *organ-preservation procedure* that is used in cases of breast cancer is a lumpectomy, which involves removing the tumor and the margins of tissue around it. After a lumpectomy, the woman usually undergoes radiation therapy to eliminate possible traces of the cancer. Until about 25 or 30 years ago, the only treatment available for breast cancer was a mastectomy, which involves removal of the entire breast and is still necessary in some cases. Depending on the size of the tumor, organ preservation is also possible for other cancers, such as those involving the head and neck, bladder, colon, and anus. Organ preservation procedures can have an extremely beneficial effect on a person's quality of life without compromising a cure.

A procedure called *second-look surgery* is performed, but rarely, to check the effect of previous surgery or possibly to remove any cancer that could not be removed during the previous surgery. This approach is sometimes used in treating ovarian cancer.

There are new approaches to destroy or ablate tumor tissue that are used by both surgeons and interventional radiologists. These approaches include *focused ultrasound* (sound waves), *cryotherapy* (cold), *radiofrequency ablation* or *RF* (radiowaves), and *phototherapy* (light) using a laser and a special chemical that makes the laser cut better. These procedures are often used in palliative situations to relieve symptoms of a tumor mass, but they are also used as the primary therapy in some instances. For some tumors in which these techniques are used, such as prostate cancer (which is a relatively slow-growing tumor), it can take many years to prove that a new local treatment such as cryotherapy or focused ultrasound has the ability to kill all of the tumor cells. While these approaches are very attractive in concept, it is important to have a good understanding of the natural history of the disease and how long a new treatment has been in use when you consider such a treatment option.

Chemotherapy

Because chemotherapy is a systemic treatment (affecting the entire body), it can be used to treat either a localized tumor or the entire body, if the tumor has metastasized. A single drug is used in some instances, but most chemotherapy regimens include a combination of three or four drugs that kill cancer cells in different ways. These drug combinations are administered according to a clearly specified schedule, or *protocol*. Because many different treatments are available, your doctor will discuss with you the regimen that is appropriate for your cancer. You won't necessarily need detailed knowledge about the drugs used in chemotherapy to make an appropriate treatment decision.

During your treatment, your oncologist will monitor your progress using the same methods that were used during the diagnostic and staging studies. The tumor's "response" will be evaluated according to the terms defined in Chapter 4.

Drug Classifications

How different anticancer drugs kill cancer cells or prevent them from dividing depends on their classification. Drugs in the same class kill the cancer cells by the same mechanism of action: that is, they all attack the same target within the cell. Most drug regimens are composed of drugs from different classes; the different drugs work in different phases of cell division (described in Chapter 2) or on different targets (some of which are described in Appendix A). For example, some drugs are incorporated into DNA and prevent cell division, others will cross-link the strands of DNA making it impossible for the cell to duplicate the DNA, others will inhibit key enzymes involved in the cell cycle or DNA synthesis, and still others may prevent the cell from undergoing mitosis by inhibiting the mitotic spindle needed to separate the chromosomes. Newer drugs work by inhibiting cell signaling pathways or by blocking the action of growth factors, as described in Chapter 7. There are other drugs that are designed to enhance the efficacy of the more standard chemotherapy agents (*modifiers* or *sensitizers*) and still others that can reduce the toxicity of treatment (*protectors*). Combination chemotherapy regimens are designed so that drugs will work in concert, making it difficult for the cancer cell to become resistant to therapy.

Some of the common chemotherapy regimens used to treat different types of cancer are listed in table 6.1. Regimens are sometimes given acronyms using the first letter of the chemical or trade name of each drug. For example, note the regimen available for Hodgkin's disease called ABVD. (The four drugs used in this regimen are listed in the table.) Doctors use these abbreviations to communicate more easily. Because the names of some different drugs begin with the same first letter, the abbreviations don't always indicate which drugs are in a particular regimen.

Table 6.1. Examples of Chemotherapy for Specific Cancer Sites

Cancer Site	Drugs	Abbreviation
Anus	5-fluorouracil (e.g., Efudex®), mitomycin (Mutamycin®)	5-FU, mitomycin
	5-fluorouracil, cisplatin (Platinol®)	5-FU, platinum
Bladder	cyclophosphamide (e.g., Cytoxan®), methotrexate, vinblastine (Velban®), (sometimes Adriamycin®)	CMV (or M-VAC)
Brain	procarbazine (Matulane®), lomustine (CeeNU®), vincristine (Oncovin®), sometimes hydroxyurea (Hydrea®)	PCV
	temozolomide (Temodar®)	
Breast	Adriamycin®, cytoxan → paclitaxel (Taxol®), and possibly Herceptin®	AC → T (possibly Herceptin®, too)
	aromatase inhibitors: anastrozole (Arimedex®), letrozole (Femara®), exemestane (Aromisin®)	
Colon or rectum	5-fluorouracil, leucovorin	5-FU, leucovorin
	fluorouracil, leucovorin, and oxaliplatin (Eloxatin®)	FOLFOX
	fluorouracil, leucovorin, and irinotecan (Campto®)	FOLFIRI
	bevacizumab (Avastin®)	
Esophagus	5-fluorouracil, cisplatin, etoposide, often with radiotherapy	
Head and neck	cisplatin, 5-fluorouracil, leucovorin, taxol, often with radiotherapy	PFL
	EGFR inhibitor	

Table 6.1. Continued

Cancer Site	Drugs	Abbreviation
Hodgkin's disease	Adriamycin®, bleomycin (Blenoxane®), vinblastine, dacarbazine	ABVD
	doxorubicin, vinblastine, mechlorethamine, vincristine, bleomycin, etoposide, and prednisone	Stanford V
	nitrogen mustard, vincristine, procarbazine plus ABVD	MOPP/ABVD hybrid
Leukemia, acute	daunorubicin (Cerubidine®), cytosine arabinoside (Cytosar®), VP-16	DA
Leukemia, chronic	chlorambucil, fludarabine (Fludara®)	
Lung	carboplatin, taxol	Carbo-taxol
	docetaxel (Taxotere®), carboplatin	
	vinorelbin, cisplatin	
	cisplatin, etoposide	
	cyclophosphamide, doxorubicin, vincristine	CAV
Lymphoma, aggressive	cyclophosphamide, doxorubicin (Adriamycin®), vincristine, prednisone, rituximab (Rituxan®)	CHOP-R
	infusional etoposide, vincristine, doxorubicin, bolus cyclophosphamide, prednisone with rituximab	EPOCH-R
Lymphoma, low-grade	cyclophosphamide, vincristine, prednisone, fludarabine (Fludara®)	CVP

Table 6.1. Continued

Cancer Site	Drugs	Abbreviation
Ovarian cancer	Cisplatin or carboplatin and taxol	
	liposomal doxorubicin (Doxil®)	
Pancreas cancer	5-flourouracil, platinum	
	gemcitabine (Gemzar®)	
Stomach cancer	5-flourouracil, leucovorin, platinum	
Testicular cancer	Cisplatin, vinblastine, bleomycin	PVB
	Cisplatin, etoposide, bleomycin	PEB
	Cisplatin, etoposide, ifosfamide	ICE

Note: In most cases, drugs are listed by their generic name, and brand names appear in parentheses.

Dosage and Scheduling

As a general rule, doctors prescribe a dosage of chemotherapy which is high enough to optimize the chance that the tumor will respond. That is why drug regimens are so carefully designed. The dosage cannot be reduced simply because the doctor or the patient doesn't like how it makes the patient feel. For the same reason, one drug cannot be arbitrarily removed from a combination regimen. Chemotherapy regimens should be modified only for reasons having to do with the effectiveness or toxicity of the treatment.

The total amount of chemotherapy administered over a specified period of time is referred to as the regimen's *dosage intensity* or *dose intensity,* whereas the *dose* is the amount of drug that is administered at one time. Individual doses of drugs are usually calculated in milligrams (mg) according to the patient's total body surface area in square meters (m^2), expressed as mg/m^2.

Another new way to calculate the correct dose, which is available for some drugs, is to combine the patient's *pharmacokinetic profile and surface area.* In this calculation, to determine how much of a drug to give to the patient, the concentration of the specific drug in the blood over time must be measured. After the patient receives the first dose of the drug, blood is taken to determine the drug's concentration; this information is then compared with pharmacokinetic information for the drug, which indicates the *effective blood concentration* that is needed for the specific drug. Subsequent doses of the drug will depend on how the patient's system handles the drug—what the blood concentration is—as well as on his or her body size. If the blood concentration is low, a bigger dose will be given, and if it is too high, the next dose will be smaller. The pharmacokinetic curve plots drug concentration (on the *y* axis) versus time (on the *x* axis). The *area under the curve* (*AUC*) is used as a measure of drug exposure. Some drugs are dosed to give patients a certain AUC. An example of a drug prescribed this way is carboplatin (Paraplatin®).

Although dosing using pharmacokinetic profile is a safer, more effective way of determining the dose an individual patient should receive, pharmacokinetic-derived dosing is currently available for only a limited number of drugs, so for many drugs it is necessary to determine doses solely on the basis of the patient's body surface and to adjust the next dose based on the toxicity (such as low blood counts).

To cure a tumor, it occasionally is necessary to use a dosage of drugs (or radiation) which may exceed the tolerance of an organ. As a result, the organ may malfunction months or years later. In some cases, the damage can be repaired with surgery: for example, by removing a damaged piece of intestine. In other cases, a drug or a hormone can replace a normal function. For instance, thyroid hormone can replace the function of a damaged thyroid gland, as it did for Betty in Chapter 3.

In general, chemotherapy is administered in cycles every three or four weeks. Patients may receive both intravenous medication and pills for 1 or 2 weeks, then recover for two weeks before the next cycle begins. The total duration of chemotherapy is usually 4 to 6 months, although some newer regimens use an intensive short-course treatment of two to three months. People with some types of leukemia need maintenance chemotherapy after their major chemotherapy ends. Maintenance chemotherapy involves drugs that are milder than those used at the beginning of treatment. These drugs are often in pill form and can be taken for months or even years.

Administration

Chemotherapy drugs can be administered either by mouth or by vein (intravenously), depending on the drug. Because drugs taken by mouth enter the bloodstream from the intestine and intravenously administered drugs enter the bloodstream directly, all of them are called *systemic therapy*.

New methods of administering chemotherapy drugs intravenously have made the treatment much easier for patients than it was in the past. For example, rather than sticking patients with a needle every time blood is withdrawn or drugs are administered, ports of access to a vein can remain in place for many months, and infusion pumps are used to administer chemotherapy to patients in the clinic and at home. One example is a *PICC* line. (PICC stands for *peripherally inserted central catheter*.) Some infusion pumps are small enough and portable enough to administer drugs continuously for a week, a month, or even longer while patients go about their normal daily activities.

Chemotherapy can be given alone, or it can be given simultaneously with radiation therapy. This is being done more commonly for head and neck, esophageal, anal, and bladder cancers. Occasionally, chemotherapy and radiation therapy are given according to an alternating schedule. As a general rule, the initial chemotherapy regimen selected is the most effective one. As you can see in table 6.1, more than one "standard" regimen is available for many cancers, and the effectiveness of all of them for a specific illness is approximately equal. For some cancers such as Hodgkin's disease, however, a doctor may initially prescribe a relatively mild drug regimen for a few months to treat a tumor mass. If the results are unsatisfactory, the doctor may then prescribe a more toxic, second-line (salvage) drug regimen. Although second-line therapies can be highly effective, doctors turn to them only when necessary because of the greater risk of late effects.

Side Effects

Almost all chemotherapy agents produce side effects that not only can affect blood counts but also can cause physical symptoms such as nausea and vomiting. Some of the possible side effects produced by different anticancer drugs are listed in table 6.2. (Table 6.4, at the end of this chapter, includes more medical terminology.) Please be assured that you are likely to experience only a few of the side effects listed there. Your doctor should carefully explain ahead of time the side effects you may experience during your specific treatment. The table is included so that you can consult it before discussing with your doctor any effects you are experiencing.

The purpose of chemotherapy is to kill cancer cells. The drugs inevitably kill normal cells, too, however. The most common side effect from chemotherapy is due to damage to *stem cells* in the bone marrow. (Stem cells are the cells that continually produce mature red cells, white cells, and platelets.) Although the stem cells that remain behind will produce new cells, some high-dosage treatments may destroy so many stem cells that they must be replaced after treatment ends by transplanting bone marrow from another person or by harvesting peripheral blood (circulating) stem cells or bone marrow stem cells from the patient before treatment begins and reinfusing the patient's own stem cells back into the patient when treatment ends. (Bone marrow transplant procedures are described at the end of this chapter.)

If the treatment poses the possibility of sterility, men can bank their sperm before treatment. First, however, it is necessary to obtain a sample to check the number of sperm and their motility. If the results are satisfactory, a few more samples are collected and frozen. With new techniques available for in vitro fertilization, even men with low sperm counts may wish to do sperm banking. Because the process of collecting sperm samples can take a week or more, it is usually done during the patient's diagnostic workup.

Table 6.2. Common Side Effects of Chemotherapy

Side Effect	Comments
Blood doesn't clot properly	Clotting factors or platelets can be administered.
Blood in the urine (hematuria)	This condition is usually temporary.
Cystitis	Irritation of the bladder. See also side effects of radiation therapy. Also a symptom of bladder cancer.
Damage to heart muscle (cardiomyopathy)	Caused by certain chemotherapeutic drugs. May be caused by the cancer itself.
Damage to liver cells (hepatic toxicity)	This condition is usually temporary but can be severe in patients undergoing bone marrow transplantation.
Difficulty urinating (dysuria)	This may occur with certain drugs.
Inflammation of the tissue lining the eyelid (conjunctivitis)	This condition is rare.
Irritation or inflammation of the skin (dermatitis)	Symptoms include rash, blisters, or sensitivity to light. These are temporary and usually clear up within a week.
Inflammation of the intestine (enteritis)	Also can be caused by an infection.
Erythema	Redness of the skin. Can also be caused by the tumor.
Fatigue	This is common but temporary.
Frequent need to empty the bladder or bowel	Usually a temporary effect.
Hair loss (alopecia)	See also side effects of radiation therapy.
Impotence	This can be temporary or permanent. It is not the same as sterility,

Table 6.2. Continued

Side Effect	Comments
	which means the inability to have children.
Inflammation or infection of the skin (cellulitis)	Can occur when blood counts are low or skin is damaged.
Inflammation of a vein (phlebitis) or a blood clot in a vein (thrombophlebitis)	Happens often in superficial veins. If a deep vein is affected, an anti-coagulant drug or surgical inter-vention may be necessary. Also can be the result of an infection.
Irritation of the rectum (proctitis)	Caused by some types of chemo-therapy. Occurs more commonly with radiation. It is generally temporary.
Itching (pruritus)	May be an allergic reaction.
Kidney damage	Usually is monitored and drug is stopped.
Liver damage	Usually is temporary but can be a serious problem in patients undergoing bone marrow trans-plantation.
Low white-blood-cell count (leukopenia)	The two major types of white blood cells are lymphocytes (lympho-penia) and granulocytes (granulo-cytopenia/neutropenia). The latter condition carries a high risk of serious infection. The risk can be reduced using cytokines and growth factors, described later in this chapter.
Loss of appetite (anorexia)	Cancer also can cause anorexia.
Loss of weight and muscle mass (cachexia)	Cancer also can cause cachexia.

Table 6.2. Continued

Side Effect	Comments
Low platelet count (thrombocytopenia)	Because platelets are essential to blood clotting, there is a risk of bleeding. Thus, drugs that reduce clotting, such as aspirin and nonsteroidal anti-inflammatory drugs, should be avoided. Platelet transfusions may be needed.
Low white-blood-cell count (lymphopenia)	The number of lymphocytes usually returns to normal.
Muscle weakness (myopathy)	In rare instances, cancer can be the cause.
Nausea or vomiting (emesis)	Emesis can be prevented by antiemetic drugs.
Nerve damage	Usually causes abnormal sensations but also can cause weakness. May be slowly reversible.
Sores or ulcers in the mouth or intestine (stomatitis)	Usually temporary. Must be distinguished from a fungal infection (thrush).
Sterility (inability to have children)	Sexual relations may still be possible. Thus, sterility is not the same as impotence.

Drug Resistance

In Chapter 2, I mentioned that cancer cells lacking an adequate blood supply are starved for oxygen. Because anticancer drugs are delivered to the tumor by the bloodstream, these *hypoxic cells* are unlikely to respond to chemotherapy (because it won't reach them through the bloodstream) until some of the tumor is eliminated. A new class of drugs which specifically kills hypoxic cells is now available. This is helpful for both chemotherapy and radiotherapy, because hypoxic cells are radioresistant.

Some cancer cells are resistant to a variety of drugs for biochemical reasons. They may lack the appropriate biochemical target, they may be able to break down the drug (*detoxify* it), or they may be able to pump the drug out of the cell before it causes any permanent harm. These cells either were resistant before treatment began or became resistant during treatment. Some cancer cells develop resistance to only one drug, and because a chemotherapy regimen usually consists of three or four drugs from different classes, cancer cells are unlikely to be resistant to at least some of them. Some cancer cells do develop resistance to drugs from several different classes, however; this is called *multiple drug resistance* or *multidrug resistance* (MDR). The causes of multiple drug resistance are currently being investigated in the laboratory, and novel therapies involving drugs or drug modifiers are being tested in clinical trials to overcome this type of chemotherapy resistance.

Radiation Therapy

Radiation therapy is delivered with powerful x-ray machines called *linear accelerators*. The energy of the x-rays these machines produce is approximately 1,000 times greater than the energy produced by the machines used for diagnostic x-ray purposes. Because the energy is so strong, the therapeutic x-rays kill tumor and normal cells.

There are a few common misconceptions about radiation therapy. For example, despite what you may have heard, people who receive standard radiation therapy are not radioactive, are not a threat to others, and don't need to give up their normal activities during therapy. The only exception is a procedure called *brachytherapy* (discussed later in this chapter). Furthermore, the radiation is not administered randomly throughout the body; it goes only where it is aimed.

Irradiated tumors tend to shrink slowly and may not disappear completely for months after treatment ends — and this is true even for tumors that are cured by radiation therapy. Therefore, the status of the tumor usually isn't checked during radiation therapy. At the appropriate time, usually starting a month after treatment, the tumor's response is evaluated by repeating the examinations and tests that were used to diagnose and stage the tumor.

Preparation

Before the actual treatment begins, the radiation oncologist, with the help of a radiation physicist and a dosage expert called a *dosimetrist,* develops a plan designed to treat the tumor and the tissues around it while minimizing damage to normal tissues within the field (or *port*) of irradiation. The planning is done with a machine called a *simulator,* which uses lower-energy, diagnostic x-rays. Simulation is often done with a CT scanner called a CT-sim.

During the simulation process, which takes about an hour, the radiation oncologist uses the results of the imaging studies described in Chapter 3 and knowledge about the natural history of the individual patient's tumor to identify the tissues that should be irradiated, including the local tumor site, regional tissue (margins and lymph nodes), and possibly a "prophylactic" site. The term *prophylactic radiation* usually refers to irradiation of a site in the body which was not initially involved with the tumor to prevent a recurrence. One example is radiation of the brain for some patients with acute leukemia to keep the disease from spreading to the tissue (meninges) that surrounds the brain.

After the necessary calculations have been made, a "block" made of lead or cerrobend is custom-designed to shape the area for therapy so that as much normal tissue as possible is spared. The block is placed on the x-ray machine before each treatment. The treatment plan and the block are then transferred to the radiation therapy department, where well-trained radiation technologists (called radiation therapists) deliver the actual treatments. X-rays called *port films* are taken at least once a week to ensure that the treatment beam and the patient's body are aligned properly. Because port films are taken using the treatment machine, the detail is unclear and the tumor cannot be observed. Therefore, these films cannot be used to measure the tumor's response.

Newer radiation therapy techniques use a computerized tomographic (CT) scanner to help define the target. Rather than using blocks, the newer linear accelerators can shape the treatment field itself using a *multileaf collimator*. Often called *3D radiotherapy* or *conformal radiotherapy*, this new technology is being used for many disease sites, especially the prostate gland, lung, and brain. The first part of the treatment may involve deeply penetrating x-rays, whereas the second part may involve electrons that penetrate only to a limited depth. The dosimetrist calculates the correct mix of x-rays and electrons.

Newer radiation therapy technology is coupled with advances in imaging using CT scans, MR images, PET scans, PET-CT scans, and others to allow increased precision. Such precision makes it possible for the radiation oncologist to deliver a higher dose to the tumor and a lower dose to normal tissues. The new technologies being used to do this include *intensity modulated radiation therapy* (*IMRT*), Tomotherapy®, Cyberknife®, Gammaknife®, *stereotactic radiotherapy* (*SRT*), and *stereotactic radiosurgery* (*SRS*). Machines that use proton beams have unique properties to finely focus the beam, which is particularly useful for small targets like brain lesions in children, for example. The use of computerized planning allows for this improved precision; therefore, it is critical to accurately locate the tumor and to minimize, or account for, patient and internal organ motion. Radiation oncologists and physicists are continually improving these techniques.

Dosage and Scheduling

The precise number of treatments will depend on the total dosage of radiation given, which the radiation oncologist determines on the basis of the type of tumor and its size, as well as the use of combined modality therapy. The term *Gray* (abbreviated *Gy*) is used to indicate the number of units in the total dosage and in individual doses. Treatment is usually given 5 days per week for 5 to 7 weeks (25 to 35 days), again depending on the type and size of the tumor. In many cases, the radiation field is relatively large during the initial treatments and later is made smaller to avoid some of the surrounding normal tissue and to zero in on the tumor (called a *cone-down field*).

The term *fractionation* describes the daily dosing schedule. For example, if the oncologist determines that a patient needs a total dosage of 60 Gy (dosages usually range from 40 to 75 Gy), the usual daily dose, or fraction, will be 1.8 to 2.0 Gy. The term *hyperfractionation* is used if a patient is scheduled to receive two doses per day for a higher total dosage of 70 to 80 Gy. In this case, each dose is reduced to 1.1 to 1.6 Gy so that less damage is produced in the normal tissues. On the other hand, *hypofractionation* is used to treat a metastasized tumor, or in some cases with a locally advanced tumor, when the patient may require a total dosage of only 30 to 40 Gy. Fewer but larger-sized fractions are used in order to reduce the time required for treatment. This patient would receive a higher daily dose of 3 to 4 Gy either 4 or 5 days per week, but usually for only 2 or 3 weeks. Shortened schedules like this are being investigated for treatment of early stage breast cancer. This treatment is called *partial breast irradiation (PBI)*.

In radiation therapy, the term *dose intensity* (total dose divided by the total number of weeks) is used to express the concept that patients with some types of tumors should receive as much radiation as possible in the shortest possible time because the effectiveness of the treatment may depend on completing the treatment before the tumor begins growing again. This type of radiation therapy is called *accelerated fractionation*. Whereas standard fractionation would deliver 70 Gy in 7 weeks, accelerated fractionation might be 70 Gy in 5 weeks.

As is true with chemotherapy, the dosage of radiation required to cure a tumor occasionally exceeds the tolerance of an organ, which may cause the organ to malfunction months or years after treatment. Usually enough of the organ is spared that the patient does not have serious side effects. In many cases methods are available to compensate for this damage, such as removing a part of the organ. In some cases, organ function will be reduced but symptoms will only appear with exertion; one example of this would be reduced lung function after lung irradiation for lung cancer.

Administration

Radiation therapy requires highly specialized equipment and up-to-date machines and techniques. Because radiation therapy is similar to surgery, in that it focuses on a specific part of the body, the radiation oncologist's skill in determining what part of the body to treat is far more important than the brand of radiation equipment used. The patient needs to rely on the radiation oncologist's expertise regarding which facility can administer the treatment most effectively and safely. The brand of machine used or whether the patient likes the facility's interior decoration or finds its location convenient are, obviously, not nearly as important as safe and effective treatment.

Side Effects

The side effects associated with radiation will depend on the part of the body which is irradiated. Some of these side effects are listed in table 6.3. (Table 6.4 at the end of this chapter includes more medical terminology.) No patient will experience all of these side effects. Your radiation oncologist and the staff will tell you about the side effects you may experience. In addition, all these details will be listed in the consent form you will be asked to sign before treatment.

Although the purpose of radiation therapy is to kill tumor cells, the treatment inevitably kills some normal cells as well. If an adequate number of stem cells remain behind in the normal tissue, they will produce new cells. For all organs, information is available about the radiation *tolerance dosage* that can be given. It is usually possible to stay below the tolerance dose; however, the need to administer a dosage of radiation which will kill the tumor cells means that late damage to normal tissue is always a risk. The dosage used and the selection of the volume of normal tissue to be treated usually produce less than a 1 to 5 percent risk of a serious late toxicity. Some of the late damage can be repaired surgically, as with damage to the intestine. In some situations a late effect may be anticipated; for example, if a man is scheduled to receive radiation therapy to his lower abdomen or pelvis, he may want to bank his sperm before treatment begins, because low sperm counts are an anticipated side effect of this treatment.

Table 6.3. Common Side Effects of Radiation Therapy

Side Effect	Comments
Blood in the urine	This is usually temporary.
Damage to the heart muscle (cardiomyopathy) or heart sac (pericardium)	Can be caused by irradiation of the heart.
Damage to the liver (hepatic toxicity)	This is usually temporary.
Difficulty urinating (dysuria)	This may occur when the pelvic area is irradiated.
Dry mouth (xerostomia)	Occurs with therapy to the mouth and salivary glands. Because xerostomia can lead to dental cavities, dental hygiene must be carefully planned.
Fatigue	This is a common side effect of treatment.
Frequent need to empty the bladder or bowel (urgency)	This is usually temporary.
Hair loss (alopecia)	Loss will be localized to the radiation field. May be permanent if high-dose radiation is used.
Impotence	This may be temporary or permanent. It is not the same as sterility, which is the inability to have children.
Inability to control urination or bowel movements (incontinence)	This can be temporary or permanent.
Inflammation of the intestines (enteritis)	Also can be caused by an infection.
Irritation of the bladder (cystitis)	This also can be a symptom of bladder cancer.
Irritation of the rectum (proctitis)	May occur with radiation to the pelvis. Although usually temporary, radiation proctitis may persist.

Table 6.3. Continued

Side Effect	Comments
Irritation or inflammation of the skin (dermatitis)	Can consist of rash, blisters, or sensitivity to light. The symptoms usually clear up within a week. Sunscreen should be used to protect irradiated skin.
Low white-blood-cell count (leucopenia)	The number of white cells returns to normal.
Sores or ulcers in the mouth or intestines (stomatitis)	Common with radiation therapy and chemotherapy. Usually heals quickly. Good nutrition is important.

Specialized Types of Radiation Therapy

In a procedure called *brachytherapy,* a radioactive implant is placed directly into a body cavity such as the uterus or into the tissue itself, such as the prostate, breast, or the head or neck. The implant can be placed temporarily (usually for 2 to 4 days) or permanently. Temporary implants can be done on an outpatient basis and require several visits to the clinic, or they can be done in the hospital over a few days. The time that visitors may spend with the patient may be restricted for safety reasons. The radioactivity in a permanent implant eventually decays until none remains. Permanent implants usually use low-energy radiation, and it is usually safe to be near the person. Patients are given specific instructions regarding visits by relatives and friends.

Radioactive molecules are used to treat some cancers. These can be given by injection or by mouth. For example, radioactive iodine is used to treat tumors involving the thyroid gland (as with Betty in Chapter 3), and radioactive strontium is used to treat cancer that has metastasized to bone.

Adjuvant Therapy

After a person's cancer has been treated successfully, the primary therapy may be followed by *adjuvant therapy* to prevent the disease from recurring; or adjuvant therapy and the treatment for the primary tumor may be delivered simultaneously. The adjuvant treatment can be chemotherapy, radiation therapy, or hormonal therapy.

One important advance in the last few decades is the finding that systemic adjuvant treatment administered to women with breast cancer after the breast is treated increases both overall survival and disease-free survival. In the case of breast cancer, choosing an appropriate adjuvant treatment for an individual patient depends on (1) the size and pathological features of her primary tumor, (2) her menopausal status, (3) the presence or absence of estrogen receptors on the cancer cells, (4) the presence or absence of malignant cells in the woman's lymph nodes and the number of nodes involved, and (5) the molecular profile of the tumor.

In the second patient story in Chapter 9, for example, Jane S. decided, after her lumpectomy, that she would not have a mastectomy. However, because one of her lymph nodes was involved, she opted to undergo adjuvant chemotherapy and radiation therapy to eliminate any remaining cancer cells in her body and thus reduce the risk that her cancer would recur.

Bone Marrow Transplantation and Peripheral Stem Cell Rescue

Some chemotherapy regimens are so intense and toxic to the bone marrow that the marrow must be reconstituted using stem cells either from the patient or from another person. Some very new treatments are taking advantage of the immune response of the donor cells against the patient's cancer to "reject" the cancer, so that the bone marrow transplantation is used as part of the anticancer treatment. This is called the "graft-versus-tumor" effect. Before the transplant, patients are hospitalized and subjected to extremely high doses of chemotherapy, and in some cases whole body radiotherapy as well. These treatments kill cancer cells but are so toxic to the bone marrow that the patients must be placed in isolation to protect them from infection.

BMT can be accomplished in one of two ways: by using the patient's own stem cells (an *autologous transplant*) or by using another person's stem cells (an *allogeneic transplant*). Either procedure can use stem cells derived from the peripheral blood or bone marrow. Bone marrow transplantation requires a harvest of bone marrow cells under general anesthesia. For an autologous transplant using peripheral stem cells, before receiving high-dose chemotherapy, the patient is injected with a growth factor that stimulates the bone marrow to produce stem cells that circulate in the bloodstream. These cells are harvested by a process called leucophoresis and are stored. After chemotherapy is completed, the cells are infused into the patient.

In the case of an allogeneic transplant, the donor is usually a close relative, such as a parent, brother, or sister (or occasionally a stranger), whose tissue, not blood type, closely matches the patient's tissue. Because the human immune system is extremely complex, finding a donor is not easy. Thus, major national and international registries contain the names of millions of people who have agreed to be potential donors (for example, the National Marrow Donor Program).

When chemotherapy ends, the donor's marrow is injected into the patient and everyone waits to see whether the graft "takes." When allogeneic BMT is successful, the donor's stem cells thrive and reproduce in the patient. Rarely the graft does not take; more commonly, even when the donor is a tissue-matched relative, the donor's immune cells may attack the patient and cause problems with the skin, liver, and intestinal tract. Called *graft-versus-host disease,* this disease is treated with drugs that suppress the immune system. As noted earlier, some cancer treatments take advantage of this graft-versus-tumor effect.

Growth Factor and Hormonal Therapy

In Chapter 2, I talked about hormones, growth factors, and cytokines that cells use to communicate by binding to receptors on the surface of other cells. These growth factors are increasingly used in standard treatment regimens and in bone marrow transplantation. Some growth factors help red blood cells, white blood cells, and platelets recover during and after chemotherapy or radiation therapy. The bone marrow growth factors in use include the colony stimulating factors G-CSF (filgrastim [Neupogen®] and pegfilgrastim [Neulasta®]) and GM-CSF (sargramostim [Leukine®]), which stimulate white blood cell production and function; thrombopoietin (TPO) and oprelviken (interleukin [IL]-11, Neumega®) which stimulate platelet production; and erythropoietin (Epogen®), which increases red blood cell production.

A few types of cancer respond to hormones in a manner that resembles the way normal tissue responds. Thus, changing the hormonal environment of a tumor may cause the tumor to shrink. For example, tumors in the breast may shrink when estrogen is removed, and tumors in the prostate gland may shrink when testosterone is removed. These sex hormones can be removed either by surgically removing their source or, more often, by blocking their effect with drugs (antihormones). Either method has minimal side effects and, when possible, is used before resorting to standard chemotherapy. For example, some studies of women with breast cancer suggest that the women who are at high risk for metastases—those who have a large local tumor or one that involves the lymph nodes—respond to drugs that block the ability of estrogen to bind to its receptors on the cancer cells. Similarly, drugs called antiandrogens, which block the effect of male hormones, are often used for men with large or biologically aggressive prostate cancer.

Table 6.4 summarizes the side effects of treatment and the medical terminology. There is a detailed scoring system called CTCAE (Common Terminology Criteria for Adverse Events), which can be found on the NCI Web site (http://ctep.cancer.gov/forms/CTCAEv3.pdf). It does not include every possible side ef-

Table 6.4. Some Side Effects of Treatment by Organ System and Medical Terminology

Organ System	Side Effect and Medical Terminology
General	Fatigue Loss of appetite (anorexia) Nausea and vomiting (emesis) Loss of weight (cachexia)
Bone marrow and immune system	Suppression of normal counts Low platelets (thrombocytopenia), Low white blood cells (leucopenia) Low infection-fighting cells (granulocytopenia) Low immune cells (lymphopenia) Low oxygen-carrying cells (anemia)
Endocrine glands Thyroid, adrenal, pituitary, ovary, testis	Decreased hormone production
Eye	Red eye (conjunctivitis) Dry eye from lacrimal gland injury Excess tearing Loss of vision or abnormal color vision (retinopathy)
Female genitals Ovary	Decreased fertility (sterility) Decreased hormone production (hot flashes) Loss of menstrual function
Vagina	Dry vagina
Gastrointestinal tract Mouth	Sores, ulcers (stomatitis) Damage to teeth and gums
Salivary glands	Dry mouth (xerostomia)
Esophagus	Difficulty swallowing (dysphagia)
Stomach	Ulceration (gastritis)

Table 6.4. Continued

Organ System	Side Effect and Medical Terminology
Intestines	Diarrhea, may have blood in it; inflammation (enteritis)
Rectum	Irritation (proctitis) Having to pass stool without much warning (rectal urgency) Loss of control of bowels (incontinence)
Heart	Muscle damage (cardiomyopathy) Inflammation to sac around heart (pericarditis) Abnormal rhythm (arrhythmia) Damage to coronary arteries
Kidney, bladder	Bladder irritation (cystitis) Uncomfortable urination (dysuria) Having to urinate frequently (frequency) Having to pass urine without much warning (urinary urgency) Blood in urine (hematuria)
Liver	Abnormal function (hepatitis or veno-occlusive disease)
Lung	Shortness of breath (dyspnea) Irritation to pleura (pleuritis) Irritation to trachea—dry cough Scarring (pulmonary fibrosis) Inflammation or infection (pneumonia or pneumonitis)
Male genitals	Decreased sperm count (infertility, sterility) Inability to have erection (impotence)
Nervous system Central—brain	Loss of concentration

Table 6.4. Continued

Organ System	Side Effect and Medical Terminology
Ear	Loss of hearing (usually high-tone loss)
	Can also be due to excess ear wax (cerumen)
Smell, taste	Abnormal or loss (usually accompanies dry mouth)
Peripheral nerves	Loss of sensation
or spinal cord	Abnormal sensation (neuropathy)
	Loss of function (paresis, or paralysis)
Skin and related structures	
Skin	Redness (erythema); infection (cellulitis); itching (pruritis); inflammation (dermatitis)
Hair	Hair loss (alopecia)
Sweat glands	Dry skin
Veins	Clot (thrombosis); or inflamed vein (phlebitis)
Soft tissue and muscle	Scarring (fibrosis); stiffness
	Muscle weakness (myopathy)

fect but has the more commonly encountered ones. The side effects will depend on the particular treatment, and most will clear up over time.

The treatments described in this chapter—both old standards and newer innovations—are available because of the work done by cancer researchers, who are working to develop new, more effective, and less toxic therapies, and patients, who agree to participate in clinical trials. The next chapter describes the emerging field of molecular-targeted therapy, and Chapter 8 details how new therapies are developed and tested and which patients might want to think seriously about getting involved in this work.

Chapter 7

Molecular-Targeted Therapy

Investments in basic research, innovative technology, and talented people to conduct research and development have ushered in the era of molecular medicine. This will impact every aspect of medicine but perhaps none as visibly and strikingly as cancer.

It has been shown that there must be abnormal function in at least four major systems for a cell to become a cancer cell. In a review describing the state of science at the beginning of the 21st century Hanahan and Weinberg used the following classification:

— Limitless replication potential
— Self-sufficiency in growth signals
— Insensitivity to antigrowth signals
— Evading apoptosis
— Tissue invasion and metastasis
— Sustained angiogenesis

They also pointed out that cancer involves both the cancer cell and the surrounding tissues, or microenvironment, including connective tissue cells, inflammatory cells, blood vessels, and other normal epithelial cells. So, cancer is a system problem (as illustrated in figure 2.1), involving the cell that undergoes mutations and also its neighbors.

As scientists learn more and more about the underlying mechanisms and pathways that make up a cancer, treatments will be developed that are selective toward the specific defect or lesion. Building on the basic knowledge presented in Chapter 2 with additional background from Appendix A, figure 7.1 illustrates the

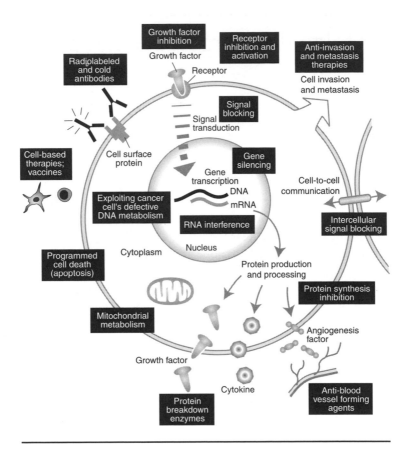

Fig. 7.1. The pathways that are potential targets for molecular-targeted cancer therapy

For each of the processes and pathways, numerous molecules can be targeted. Many new molecular-targeted drugs are being developed in the laboratory, and clinical trials conducted by translational researchers are bringing these drugs to patients. To best understand the results in patients tissue samples must be obtained before, during, and after treatment.

concept behind molecular-targeted cancer treatment. To bring laboratory advances ("the bench") to patients ("the clinic" or "the bedside"), requires physician-scientists who are knowledgeable about basic science and clinical investigation. This bench-to-bedside research is called *translational research*.

Figure 7.1 illustrates some of the general pathways that are potential targets for molecular-targeted therapy. A few points are noteworthy:

— There are multiple ways a pathway can be defective, so it may be necessary to use a few drugs to effectively hit the same pathway.
— The pathways in a cell are a complex network, so changing one pathway can have many effects. Molecular biology techniques such as *genomics, microarrays,* and *proteomics* (see Appendix A) help scientists define the multiple defects and changes that occur in a cancer.
— Molecular-targeted drugs may not necessarily kill the cells by themselves, so to be most effective they may be used in combination with conventional chemotherapy and radiation therapy.
— The target may be the cancer cell but may also be the normal tissue component within the cancer. Examples of this include supporting cells (called *stromal* cells), immune cells, or blood vessels. (The stromal cells and inflammatory cells produce growth factors that allow the malignant cell to grow and invade.)
— Novel imaging techniques called molecular imaging are being developed. Molecular imaging involves all the available standard technologies, novel imaging agents, new sequences for using the standard imaging technologies, and completely new technologies such as *nanotechnology*. Nanotechnology involves very tiny objects or devices that may be used for imaging, drug delivery, and someday may even be able to help restore or repair tissue.

Table 7.1 lists some of the molecular-targeted therapies currently in use. Some of these therapies are still under investigation,

Table 7.1. Examples of Molecular-Targeted Therapy

Molecular Target	Therapy	Type of Cancer Treated in Clinical Trials
Antibody, cold (not radioactive)	Anti-Her 2: trastuzumab (Herceptin®)	Breast cancer
	Anti-CD20: rituximab (Rituxin®)	Lymphoma
Antibody, radiolabeled	Anti-CD20: tositumomab (Bexxar®); ibritumomab tiuxetan (Zevalin®)	Lymphoma
Growth factor receptor antibody	Epidermal growth factor receptor (EGFR): cetuximab, C225 (Erbitux®)	Lung cancer, head and neck cancer
Growth factor receptor activation—metabolic inhibitor	EGFR-ZD1836: gefitinib (Iressa®); erlotinib (Tarceva®)	Lung cancer, head and neck cancer, other cancers
Growth factor inhibitors and multi-targets	VEGF inhibitor: sorafenib (BAY 43–9006)	Renal cell cancer
Signal transduction	imatinib (Gleevec®)	Chronic myelogenous leukemia, gastrointestinal stromal tumors (GIST)
	mTOR inhibitors: temsirolimus (CCI-779)	Breast cancer, lymphoma
Protein location and trafficking	Farnesyl transferase inhibitors: tipifarnib (Zarnestra®); lonafarnib (Sarasar®)	Lung cancer, breast cancer, leukemia
Protein trafficking	geldanamycin (17-AAG)	Breast cancer, melanoma
Protein breakdown	PS341; bortezomib (Velcade®)	Multiple myeloma

Table 7.1. Continued

Molecular Target	Therapy	Type of Cancer Treated in Clinical Trials
Cell cycle inhibitors	CDK (cyclin dependent kinase) inhibitors: flavopiridol, staurosporine, UCN-01	Lymphoma
Anti-angiogenic (anti–blood vessel) agents	thalidomide	Multiple myeloma
	bevacizumab (Avastin®)	Colorectal cancer
Anti-invasion and metastasis	Matrix metalloproteinase inhibitors: marmistat	
Gene silencing	Methylation: azacytidine (Vidaza®); histone acetylation: HDAC inhibitors, depsipeptide, SAHA	Myelodysplastic syndrome
Vaccines for treatment	PSA vaccine; CEA vaccine, CEA-TRICOM	Prostate cancer, gastrointestinal cancer
Vaccine for disease prevention	HPV vaccine	Cervical cancer
Chemoprevention; anti-inflammation	COX inhibitors	

while others have already been approved by the FDA. This is only a partial list and it will, of course, change dramatically over the coming years. If you wish to learn more about a specific drug, this NCI Web site may be helpful: www.nci.nih.gov/drugdictionary/. More general information on cancer treatment can be found at www.nci.nih.gov/cancertopics.

As you can see, approaches to cancer are changing dramatically due to use of molecular biology techniques, biomarkers, novel imaging, molecular signatures and profiling, and molecular-targeted therapy, which is usually used in conjunction with the more standard therapies. To access many of these new treatments early on means you must participate in a clinical trial. Clinical trials are described in Chapter 8.

Clinical Research Trials:
What They're All About

To provide better treatments tomorrow than we have today, advances in knowledge are necessary. All advances in the treatment of cancer come from carefully conducted clinical trials. Clinical trials provide well-thought-out treatments and are designed to help oncologists develop superior treatments. This chapter explains the details involved in clinical trials and the importance given to clinical trials in health care policy.

Much of the information used by doctors in making decisions comes either from their own personal experience in treating patients or from the experience of a group of doctors in a medical center who "looked back" at patients they had treated and published an article about treatment outcomes in a medical journal. Both of these sources of information are considered *retrospective trials,* and they are useful to some extent. However, the most valuable information comes from *prospective clinical trials,* which are carefully designed by physicians and statisticians to answer a specific question. As we are now in the era of evidence-based medicine, decision making and reimbursement will depend more and more on data from prospective clinical trials.

Prospective clinical trials fall into two general categories: *developmental trials* and *comparative randomized trials.* In developmental clinical trials, also called Phase I and Phase II trials, new treatments developed in the laboratory are tested in small groups of patients. Because a new treatment may have more side effects than an older treatment does, it must be investigated with great care. If the results look promising, the new treatment is tested in a *comparative randomized trial,* which usually involves a large number of patients. Also called Phase III trials, comparative randomized trials are the best way to tell with certainty whether a new treatment is better than an older one.

Phase I and Phase II Clinical Trials

A Phase I trial is designed to determine the proper dosage and dosing schedule for a new treatment and to define its side effects. The initial dosage is selected according to the results of laboratory research. In Phase I trials, the type of cancer is usually not important; thus, patients with a variety of malignancies receive the same treatment. As more patients enter the study, the dosage is carefully increased. Although Phase I trials are not conducted to investigate whether a new treatment is effective, the tumors of the participants in these trials may have an excellent response. Depending on the results of the trial, investigators will proceed to conduct a Phase II trial.

The purpose of Phase II clinical trials is to determine whether the new treatment shrinks a specific type of tumor. To test its effectiveness, the treatment is given to a small group of approximately 30 patients who have the same disease. When the trial is completed, which usually takes about a year, the results are compared with the results of the standard treatment reported in the medical literature or with the results in a group of patients who in the past have received the standard treatment at the institution where the Phase II trial has been conducted. These comparison groups are called historical controls. Because only a limited number of patients participate in a Phase II trial, the rate of response may be somewhat inaccurate and therefore is not used to predict the overall response rate. The new treatment may prove to be an important advance, or it may be no better than the standard treatment; the only way to find out is to compare the two treatments in a Phase III trial. In the era of molecular medicine, responses are often assessed using biomarkers or imaging in addition to the more standard response criteria described below.

Level of Evidence for Clinical Trials

In the era of evidence-based medicine, treatment recommendations are made based on evidence from clinical trials and peer review reports. Trials vary by study design, number of patients, and endpoints. Studies can be ranked in order of how useful the results will be for determining whether a new treatment is acceptable or when a new drug will be approved for clinical use. In the steps from new science to routine, reimbursed clinical care, different types of trials are necessary. The following outline from the NCI Physician Data Query (PDQ) Web site (www.nci.nih.gov/cancertopics/pdq/levels-evidence-adult-treatment) is included to give you a general framework for how decisions about bringing new treatments into medical care are made.

I. Strength of Study Design (in descending order of strength):
   1. Randomized controlled clinical trials
      i. Double-blinded (Treatment is determined by computer. Neither the patient not the physician know if the patient is receiving the treatment or a placebo.)
      ii. Nonblinded (Treatment is determined by a computer. The patient and the physician know whether the patient is receiving the treatment or a placebo.)
   2. Nonrandomized controlled clinical trials
   3. Case series
II. Strength of Endpoints (in descending order of strength):
   1. Total mortality (or overall survival from a defined time)
   2. Cause-specific mortality (or cause-specific mortality from a defined time)
   3. Carefully assessed quality of life
   4. Indirect surrogates
      i. Disease-free survival
      ii. Progression-free survival
      iii. Tumor response rate

The system for recommendations and ratings for clinical application of medical treatments used by the U.S. Preventive Services Task Force (USPSTF) follows. These are available on the Agency for Healthcare

Research and Quality (AHRQ) Web site (www.ahrq.gov/clinic/ajpm suppl/harris3.htm).

USPSTF Recommendations and Ratings

The USPSTF grades its recommendations for use of medical treatments according to one of five classifications (A, B, C, D, or I) that reflect the strength of evidence and magnitude of net benefit (benefits minus harms) of the study used to determine the recommendation:

A The USPSTF strongly recommends that clinicians provide [the service] to eligible patients. The USPSTF found good evidence that [the service] improves important health outcomes and concludes that benefits substantially outweigh harms.

B The USPSTF recommends that clinicians provide [the service] to eligible patients. The USPSTF found at least fair evidence that [the service] improves important health outcomes and concludes that benefits outweigh harms.

C The USPSTF makes no recommendation for or against routine provision of [the service]. The USPSTF found at least fair evidence that [the service] can improve health outcomes but concludes that the balance of benefits and harms is too close to justify a general recommendation.

D The USPSTF recommends against routinely providing [the service] to asymptomatic patients. The USPSTF found at least fair evidence that [the service] is ineffective or that harms outweigh benefits.

I The USPSTF concludes that the evidence is insufficient to recommend for or against routinely providing [the service]. Evidence that [the service] is effective is lacking, of poor quality, or conflicting, and the balance of benefits and harms cannot be determined.

Using a system similar to that of PDQ, the U.S. Preventive Services Task Force rating of evidence is (in descending order of strength):

• Level I: Evidence obtained from at least one properly designed randomized controlled trial.
• Level II-1: Evidence obtained from well-designed controlled trials without randomization.

- Level II-2: Evidence obtained from well-designed cohort or case-control analytic studies, preferably from more than one center or research group. (These trials have specific methodology, the details of which are not important to this discussion.)
- Level II-3: Evidence obtained from multiple time series with or without the intervention. Dramatic results in uncontrolled trials could also be regarded as this type of evidence.
- Level III: Opinions of respected authorities, based on clinical experience, descriptive studies, or reports of expert committees.

The increased use of clinical trials results to determine treatment policy and reimbursement emphasizes the importance given to knowledge obtained from well-designed clinical trials.

Phase III Clinical Trials

When a Phase III trial is planned, many steps are usually involved. First, a group of investigators, under the leadership of a principal investigator, decides what question the research should be designed to answer. Members of the group write down their ideas on a document called a *Concept Sheet*, which is reviewed by a Scientific Review Committee composed of members of the institution that will bear primary responsibility for the research. More and more, patient advocates are participating in the planning of clinical trials. This institution can be a hospital, a cancer center, or a national Cooperative Group made up of doctors, statisticians, and data managers from multiple institutions with funding from the National Cancer Institute. Some Phase III trials (and Phase IV "after-market" trials) are sponsored by pharmaceutical companies. Because most Phase III trials include many hundreds of patients and involve a tremendous amount of time, effort, and money, a number of major institutions and community practices usually participate. The investigators and committees work hard to ensure that the question being asked in the trial is an important one and that the study is well designed to answer it. For multicenter trials supported by the NCI, Data Safety and Monitoring Boards (DSMBs) are required to provide an additional level of oversight. They look at interim analyses of the trial and close the study if one of the arms of the trial is superior to the other or if there is undue toxicity.

Biomarkers, Intermediate Markers, and Surrogate Endpoints

Accompanying the revolution in molecular biology and molecular-targeted therapy are new clinical trial designs. Many of the new molecular therapies described in Chapter 7 do not kill the cancer cells by themselves but require the use of conventional chemotherapy and radiation therapy. So, there are two ways of judging efficacy. The first is to test a standard treatment alone compared to the standard treatment plus the new therapy, studying the conventional endpoints: survival, freedom from relapse, response rate, and so on. However, since the new drug acts against a molecular target (that's why it is called molecular-targeted therapy), there is an interest in studying the specific molecular target in the patient before, during, and after drug administration. For example, if the epidermal growth factor receptor (EGFR) is the target, is it present on the tumor cell before treatment? Does the function of the receptor change after treatment (as studied by molecular biology techniques)? Does the molecular structure of the target determine if the drug will work? (The drug may or may not work with specific mutations.) If the treatment stops working, why does it stop working? What changed in the molecular biology?

A molecular process that corresponds with the disease activity or the efficacy of treatment is called a biomarker. Prostate specific antigen (PSA), is a biomarker for the presence of prostate cancer. A change in the concentration of a molecule following therapy — for example, a decrease in the amount of the angiogenesis (blood vessel production) factor vascular endothelial growth factor (VEGF) in the blood may be a marker of an effective anti-angiogenesis treatment. The change in activation state of the EGFR may be a biomarker for the efficacy of an EGFR inhibitor.

So, biomarkers are useful to scientists and physicians in understanding whether and how a drug is working.

Clinical trials are evolving to use biomarkers as the *surrogate endpoints* that predict for the more conventional endpoints such as survival and freedom from relapse. Other surrogate endpoints being developed involve imaging. Can the change in an MR or PET scan predict clinical outcome? In some cases, it appears so. Of course, for a surrogate marker to be useful it must accurately predict the clinical outcome. Consequently, a good deal of research work is required to validate the surrogate endpoint. Surrogate endpoints are also referred to as *intermediate markers*, because they can predict a clinical outcome earlier in the trial. Once the surrogate market is demonstrated to accurately predict clinical outcome (what happens to the patient), the surrogate marker is said to be validated and can become the final endpoint. In such a setting, it may be possible to do trials more rapidly and require fewer patients. This would accelerate the processes of discovery and bringing new science and new treatments into clinical use.

So, while the purpose of clinical trials remains the same — to develop evidence that will change the management of an illness — the means to get these results is evolving with biomarkers, surrogate endpoints, and innovative trial design.

Pharmacokinetic Endpoints

For some drugs there is a known relationship between the pharmacokinetic profile and efficacy or toxicity. The pharmacokinetic profile is determined by measuring the concentration of the drug in the blood over time and looking at the curves of the profile. These curves may correspond to drug efficacy or toxicity, as described in Chapter 6.

Some of the newer molecular-targeted drugs may have no toxicity, little efficacy by themselves, and no good biomarkers. What may be known is the concentration of drug needed to produce the desired molecular effect in the laboratory. For these drugs, the trial may be designed to see whether or not that concentration can be achieved in people and, if so, that is the endpoint. The amount of drug needed to produce the desired concentration will then be used to study the new drug in combination with the standard radiation or chemotherapy.

The Formal Research Protocol

Once the research concept is approved, the investigators develop a formal research protocol—a detailed, written description of the purpose of the research, who will be eligible to participate, how many patients will be needed to make the research statistically valuable, and so forth. (The specific components of a research protocol for a Phase III clinical trial appear below.)

The Components of a Clinical Research Protocol

Background. This section describes the reason for conducting the study.

Treatment regimens. Describes in great detail the treatment or treatments that the participants will undergo.

Eligibility criteria. These criteria clearly indicate who is eligible to participate in the trial. They specify the site of the cancer, its stage, its histological characteristics, the results of the person's blood tests, the person's functional (performance) status, previous treatments, and so forth.

Ineligibility criteria. These criteria clearly indicate who will be excluded from participating in the trial; in other words, people who fail to meet the eligibility criteria because the new treatment may be too toxic for them.

Pretreatment tests. The laboratory and imaging tests that will be performed before treatment begins.

Allowable modifications of the dosage and dosing schedule. Rules concerning how the treatment should be modified if blood counts decline or if other side effects develop during treatment.

Follow-up schedule. A firm schedule regarding when laboratory tests and imaging studies must be performed to monitor the effects of the treatment throughout the trial and after the trial is completed. The criteria to be used to judge response and toxicity are clearly defined.

Statistical analysis. An evaluation by an expert in biostatistics stating that the study has been properly designed.

Consent form. A form participants sign giving the medical center permission to administer a treatment. It includes the possible side effects of the treatment. To ensure that the risks and benefits of the treatment are clearly explained and that no unnecessary risks are taken, the form is reviewed and approved by a committee of experts and people from the community called an Institutional Review Board (IRB). The form is also referred to as "informed consent."

The protocol is then approved by the Institutional Review Boards and statistical experts at all the participating institutions. If the study involves a Cooperative Group, the specialty committees of the group also must approve the protocol. Patient advocates are often included in the protocol review process so that the patients' point of view is represented. Many studies are also reviewed by the National Cancer Institute. When all the participating investigators and committees have reviewed the protocol and offered their suggestions and recommendations, the principal investigator puts the protocol into final form and again obtains the approval of all the committees involved. Because the details of the treatment are precisely defined in the protocol, all participants receive high-quality treatment. Every effort is made to protect participants from injury through careful preclinical testing before the trial and through supervision by oversight committees during the trial.

Phase III clinical trials can take several years to complete. Each year (or more frequently) during the trial, the Institutional Review Boards, the DSMB, and statisticians review the research to ensure that the investigators are following the rules specified in the protocol and that the levels of toxicity are acceptable. All studies have a "stopping rule," which specifies that during the periodic reviews, the statisticians will analyze the study to see if it may have answered the question earlier than expected. If it has, the study is stopped.

Selection of Patients

To achieve a statistically valid comparison of the two treatments, two or sometimes more large groups of people with the same type and stage of cancer must be entered into the trial: an experimental group that receives the new therapy, and a control group that receives the standard therapy. In some studies, the people in the control group do not receive treatment. However, these people already will have received a standard treatment for their disease. For example, the study may ask if 6 months of treatment are enough, so at 6 months half the patients stop treatment and the others continue for a set period of time.

To avoid an imbalance of participants in each group, a statistician uses a computer to assign the participants at random to the treatment group or the control group in a manner resembling the toss of a coin. Thus, both groups are composed of a similar mix of patients with regard to characteristics such as age and general health. Consequently, any differences in the effectiveness or toxicity of the treatments will be the result of the treatments themselves rather than the result of an imbalance caused by having more elderly or ill people in one group or the other.

Experimental Treatments

Clinical trials are currently under way to assess preventive therapies as well as new approaches to treatment. There is every reason to believe that the results of some of these trials will improve the effectiveness of cancer treatment and prevent some cancers from occurring in the first place. Here are some of the promising developments that are being investigated for cancer or which may soon be investigated. Molecular-targeted therapy was discussed in Chapter 7.

Adjuvant Therapy

Beginning in the 1970s, clinical trials involving women with breast cancer demonstrated the advantage of using adjuvant chemotherapy after mastectomy in premenopausal women whose lymph nodes were involved in the cancer. Adjuvant therapy can be either chemotherapy or hormonal therapy that is given to patients who have no apparent residual cancer, with the intent of eradicating microscopic disease and thereby preventing a relapse. More recent trials have indicated that adjuvant therapy is beneficial even when the lymph nodes are not involved. Adjuvant therapy has also been effective with other diseases, including colon, lung, and prostate cancers.

For some tumors, the chemotherapy is given before the surgery or radiation therapy rather than afterward. This is referred to as *neoadjuvant chemotherapy*. The idea in neoadjuvant therapy is that it not only may eliminate any tumor cells that have migrated to other parts of the body but also may shrink the primary tumor so that it can be treated more easily with surgery or radiation therapy.

Preventive Therapy

Obviously, preventing cancers from developing in the first place would be ideal. Often referred to as *chemoprevention*, this treatment is different from chemotherapy. Trials involving chemopreventive therapy require extremely large numbers of people who are at high risk for the disease because of their family history, exposure, or the presence of a mutated gene. The chemopreventive agent must have very minimal side effects, since it is given to many people, none of whom have cancer. People who are at very high risk for a disease such as breast or colon cancer will also undergo frequent surveillance studies (mammograms for breast cancer and colonoscopy for colon tumors). Some may choose to have a breast or section of colon removed to reduce their risk. The impact of this prophylactic organ removal on the prevention of a cancer is complex, as it may be a big tradeoff to lose an organ such as a breast or an ovary for a small improvement in survival. This is an ongoing issue for women who have breast cancer suscepti-bility genes such as BRCA1 and BRCA2.

New Approaches

Technical devices. New technical devices are constantly being developed, including minimally invasive surgery, the use of heat, cold, or ultrasound to kill cancers, and other approaches. (These were discussed in Chapter 6.) These devices must be developed in conjunction with the Food and Drug Administration (FDA) to assure safety.

Modifiers (sensitizers and protectors). Drugs called modifiers can be used to alter the effectiveness of standard chemotherapy or radiation therapy. There are two kinds of modifiers: sensitizers and protectors. Unlike chemotherapy and radiation, modifiers do not kill the tumor; those called *sensitizers* make the standard treat-ment more effective, and those called *protectors* make the standard treatment less toxic. For a modifier to be useful, it must affect the tumor and normal tissue differently. If a sensitizer increased the ability of the standard treatment to kill tumor cells and nor-mal cells to the same extent, it would be no different than simply giving a higher dosage of chemotherapy or radiotherapy. The new area of molecular-targeted therapy is described in Chapter 7.

Immunotherapy. The broad category of biological therapies in-volves a wide array of approaches. One of them kills cancer cells directly by using components of the body's immune system, in-cluding molecules (cytokines, lymphokines, or interleukins) that cells use to communicate with one another. Another uses white blood cells (lymphocytes) that are specifically engineered to kill tumor cells, and a third uses monoclonal antibodies that either kill tumor cells directly or carry a poisonous substance or a radioac-tive particle to the tumor cell.

Gene therapy. There are two major concepts in gene therapy. The first involves replacing a defective gene in a cell so that the cell does not become cancerous. Because all the cells in the person's body or in the cancer would need the new gene, this procedure would be extremely complicated in cancer therapy. Although this approach is just being readied for use in clinical trials involving patients with cancer, it is being tested in preventing some hereditary metabolic diseases.

The second concept is to introduce a gene that produces a toxin that kills the cancer cells. One example being used in the clinic involves placing a gene into some of the tumor cells. The gene tells the cells to produce an enzyme that will turn a nontoxic drug into a toxic one. This "activated" drug will then diffuse to the surrounding cancer cells and kill them. In a similar manner, the gene can be placed into lymphocytes (white blood cells) or other cells, which are then injected into the patient, sometimes directly into the tumor. The lymphocyte chosen is one that homes in on the tumor, where the gene therapy can either produce a toxin or activate a drug that kills the cancer cells.

Antisense therapy. As described in Chapter 2, an oncogene may produce a defective product. In antisense therapy, a gene or a segment of DNA is introduced into the tumor cell to prevent the oncogene from making its product. The use of RNAi (*RNA interference*) to silence genes is under development (Appendix A).

Participating in a Clinical Trial: Is It for You?

Should you participate in a clinical research trial? Before making a decision, you need to consider both the pros and the cons—both the positive and the negative factors involved.

Positive Aspects

The positive aspects of participating in a clinical trial are as follows. First, the medical community gains knowledge from the information obtained in clinical trials, and this knowledge can be used to treat patients as well as to design even newer treatments. Patients benefit, too, because they receive a carefully designed regimen of treatment that is either the best standard treatment available or a new treatment that may become the best standard treatment available in the future. In fact, some cancer therapies are available only in clinical trials.

Second, despite what you may have heard, people who participate in these trials are not "guinea pigs." As I have already mentioned, the trials conducted by major cancer centers, Cooperative Groups, and the National Cancer Institute are carefully designed, and the results are painstakingly analyzed. Thus, whether you are assigned to an experimental group or a control group, you will receive excellent treatment.

Third, many of the standard treatments that your doctors will recommend have been tested in Phase III trials. Most improvements in treatment are small ones that can be detected only by conducting such trials. The greater the number of patients who choose to participate, the sooner the questions can be answered, and more patients can benefit.

Fourth, in some cases, the best treatment may be available only in a clinical research study. For example, Mary B., whose case is described in the next chapter, discovered that she had a brain tumor that could not be removed surgically. After discussing her treatment options, which could not cure her but could give her some extra months of life, she decided to participate in a Phase II clinical trial that was investigating the results of simultaneous radiation therapy and chemotherapy, followed by adjuvant chemotherapy. This treatment option was not available to Mary except through the clinical trial.

Fifth, because the treatment regimens are carefully designed and the rules described in the protocol are strict, participants receive the correct dosage of treatment. The correct dosage is extremely important because a good treatment regimen may not work well if the dosage is incorrect.

Sixth, all protocols contain "stopping rules": If one treatment definitely proves to be superior to the other treatment, the study is stopped. Therefore, no patient intentionally receives an inferior treatment.

There are other, less obvious benefits to participating in clinical research. As part of my research program, I have been involved in Phase I, II, and III trials for many years, and I have found that, aside from deriving direct benefits from the treatment, many patients feel good about contributing to medical knowledge. In addition to hoping that a novel treatment would benefit her, Mary B.

hoped that by participating in a research study she might provide new information that would benefit future patients.

Negative Aspects

Clinical trials are not available for all cancers, and those that are available are not for everyone. Good standard therapies are available for many cancers. For some cancers, however, no available treatments are particularly effective, and there may not be any great new ideas ready for testing in clinical trials.

As noted above, patients who participate in Phase III trials are assigned at random to the experimental or control group. Some people are simply not comfortable with this process and want just one recommendation from their doctor. In reality, it turns out that only a small percentage of patients who are eligible to participate in a specific clinical trial are actually entered. If a clinical trial is available and a person is eligible and is willing to participate in it, the doctor is obligated to explain and discuss all the treatment options as thoroughly as possible before the person agrees to participate. A person should never feel pressured to participate in a trial.

Medical Breakthroughs

Patients, doctors, scientists, journalists, congressional representatives, and everyone else await scientific breakthroughs. Media reports of scientific advances are simultaneously exciting and possibly misleading. Our society is hungry for news, and the hype surrounding news reports may not be helpful to people with cancer and their families. New discoveries can be made rapidly in the controlled conditions of a *laboratory experiment*. However, *clinical advances* (which directly affect patient care) are made slowly and, usually, "by inches."

Many of my patients come in to see me with newspaper and magazine clippings and Internet printouts touting a miracle cure, or articles from medical journals reporting on a new treatment regimen. At great personal and family expense people often seek a treatment that, in truth, is no better than a standard treatment.

Many people with a cancer for which the state-of-the-art treatment is not likely to be successful, understandably, become desperate. But the premature presentation of a new technical development or a scientific discovery — either by the popular media or in medical and scientific journals — is unfortunate, because it can generate unwarranted hope. Careful clinical research is required to prove that one treatment is superior to another. To quote one of my colleagues regarding new treatments, we should "test it, not tout it."

Articles submitted to medical journals are carefully reviewed by experts in the relevant field before they are published, and articles published in these peer-reviewed journals generally present reliable information. However, even peer-reviewed articles can be more optimistic than realistic. If articles in medical journals sound interesting, I encourage you to investigate them carefully. However, do not place too much stock in news reports, information on the Internet, or press releases without talking with your doctor first.

Many important advances in treatment have resulted from clinical trials, and many of today's treatments are available as a direct result of clinical research. But many questions remain to be answered — questions such as the following:

— Which chemotherapeutic regimen is best for each cancer?
— What is the proper timing of radiation therapy and adjuvant therapy?
— What are the possible late effects of a specific treatment?
— Can late effects be minimized by modifying the treatment?
— Are completely novel treatments available which may be effective, whereas standard treatments are not effective?

Crucially important questions such as these are being addressed in a number of major national and international clinical trials sponsored by Cooperative Groups and the National Cancer Institute.

If you are interested in participating in a clinical research study, your doctor or cancer center may be able to tell you about appropriate trials that are available. If not, the best place to find out is from the National Cancer Institute's PDQ—Physicians Data Query, which includes up-to-date information about treatments that are acceptable for different cancers as well as about ongoing clinical trials (for more information about PDQ, see Chapter 1).

Chapter 9

Clinical Case Studies:
Four Patient Stories

The four patient stories in this chapter are designed to help you become more familiar with how decisions about treatment are made. Each case follows the organization of the Patient's Checklist presented in Chapter 1. (A copy of the checklist for your use is presented in Appendix D.)

Each of the patients in these stories has a different type of cancer. The cancers represented are (1) non-Hodgkin's lymphoma, (2) early breast cancer, (3) early prostate cancer, and (4) a brain tumor. The patients are not real people, so please do not assume, if a case involves a medical problem that is similar to yours, that the treatment recommendations will be suitable for you. My intention is to illustrate two things: (1) the information that is included in a typical Patient's Checklist and (2) the variety of situations that arise for people with cancer. I do not intend my presentation of these cases to be interpreted as recommending any specific treatment regimens.

These case studies do not include every option available, but they will give you an idea of how someone might go about deciding among the major treatment options. My hope is that reading through at least one case study will enable you to practice the decision-making process yourself and to feel more comfortable about approaching your own situation.

Case Study 1

Bob G.'s story illustrates the importance of molecular pathology in determining the treatment approach to lymphomas. It also describes the use of new treatment using monoclonal antibodies, molecular profiling of the individual's tumor, and the need for long-term follow-up.

Medical History

Bob G. is a 63-year-old man who had been going through a tough 8 or so years. He had been happily married to his college sweetheart Adrienne since age 25, and they had two children now in their 30s. Adrienne was tragically injured in a motor vehicle accident caused by a drunk driver. After they worked hard on her rehabilitation for a year (which was not particularly successful), Bob's wife developed pneumonia and passed away. An accountant, Bob was always a bit of an anxious man and frequently used antacids. The stress of his wife's illness was very difficult for him and his family but they pulled together, and 6 years ago, the youngest child graduated from college. At the wedding of his oldest son 4 years ago, Bob ran into the sister of an old family friend. Holly was in her early 50s, had been divorced for 10 years, and had two children in their late teens. Bob and Holly ended up getting married. The blended families worked well but Bob now had two more children to worry about, and with his constantly upset stomach, he was put on drugs called *proton-pump blockers* to help reduce stomach acid.

Despite being on this medicine for 3 years, Bob frequently had an upset stomach. This was getting more annoying to him, so his doctor decided that he should see a gastroenterologist for endoscopy. The endoscopy revealed that the walls of Bob's stomach were thickened and a bit reddened, but no ulcer was seen. A small biopsy was taken and a few days later the pathology report came back, indicating that Bob had non-Hodgkin's lymphoma. His gastroenterologist felt that Bob should see a general surgeon and a medical oncologist-hematologist in his practice group.

Diagnosis

As Bob and his family were about to find out, non-Hodgkin's lymphoma encompasses a bewildering list of subtypes. There are two widely used classification schemes: the Working Formulation and the Revised European American Lymphoma (REAL) classification. The pathologist who examined the slides said that Bob's biopsy was not a very big piece of tissue, which is often the case, and that the cells she saw were a mixture of large and small lymphocytes. She favored the diagnosis of large cell lymphoma, possibly the result of a conversion from a long-standing small cell lymphoma, but felt that the tissue sample needed to be sent to a major cancer center for review, and possibly further study. She thought that a bigger sample might be needed for special molecular biology studies, but she decided to wait until the lymphoma pathologist saw it.

While the sample was being reviewed, Bob saw a surgeon who told him that surgery is not generally indicated for lymphoma. It is very hard to get around the entire mass because the margins of the tumor are hard to define, so to do so would be very extensive surgery and might not be successful. But even more important is that lymphomas can be successfully treated with chemotherapy and radiation therapy without requiring surgery. If Bob had any problems that might need the surgeon's help, such as serious bleeding or a perforation (hole in the stomach) during treatment, the surgeon would be available, but these problems are very rare.

The pathology slides were reviewed by a world-renowned lymphoma pathologist at an NCI-designated cancer center. She suspected that Bob's was a large cell lymphoma, but the biopsy was a very small piece and there was no extra tissue from the biopsy that could be used for immunohistological molecular biology studies. She recommended that Bob have another biopsy done and that the fresh tissue be sent to her laboratory for special studies, including molecular profiling of the tissue. Bob had seen an oncologist, who agreed that it was critical to have the right diagnosis as treatments vary widely based on the subtype of the lymphoma. So, Bob, already anxious, agreed to do this right away.

A week after the second biopsy was done, the complete analysis was finished. The pathologist diagnosed diffuse large cell lymphoma, B-cell type. The surface of the tumor cells had molecular markers of B-cell lymphoma, including one called *CD-20 (CD* stands for *cluster of differentiation*). There were some smaller lymphocytes within the biopsy specimen, suggesting that this may have started as a small cell lymphoma and progressed to a more aggressive large cell type. The tissue was also stained for a bacteria called H. pylori, because this kind of bacterial infection can be an initial cause of lymphoma. The test was negative (no bacteria was seen).

Staging Studies

The physical examination was normal. Lymph nodes are normally present in many regions of the body and those that could be felt, such as under the armpit (*axilla*) and in the groin (*inguinal region*), were normal. The liver and spleen were not enlarged on physical exam. A careful head and neck examination was done, looking at lymph node groups in the tonsils, tongue, and around the jaw, and these were normal. The results of blood studies were all normal except for the lactate dehydrogenase (LDH) level, which was elevated at two times the normal level.

CT scans were done of Bob's entire body. His stomach appeared normal, except for thickening of about one-quarter of the stomach suggesting involvement by lymphoma. No lymph nodes in the abdomen looked enlarged, although some near the stomach were on the borderline of normal size. An FDG-PET scan was done that was abnormal in the stomach but nowhere else. Bob's lymphoma was classified as *clinical stage IEA* (CS IEA). The Roman numeral "I" means that there is a single site of involvement, meaning that only one organ is affected; "E" stands for a site with no lymph nodes — called an *extranodal site* — because the cancer is in Bob's stomach rather than a nodal site such as the axilla or groin area. A nodal site would be "N." Bob has an "A," which means systemic symptoms of fever and weight loss are absent. If symptoms were present, it would be "B."

Pathologic Staging

Additional tissue was sampled to determine the final stage of disease. Bob also had a bone marrow biopsy, because it is known that lymphomas can spread to the bone marrow. This showed a few clusters of small lymphocytes in the marrow, but because they were not characteristic of lymphoma, the test results were considered negative. So Bob's cancer is now CS IEA and PS IEA.

The oncologist then told Bob and his family about the International Prognostic Index (IPI) for aggressive non-Hodgkin's lymphoma (diffuse large cell lymphoma), which identifies five significant risk factors that help predict overall survival:

1. Age (≤60 years of age vs. >60 years of age).
2. Serum lactate dehydrogenase (LDH) (normal vs. elevated).
3. Performance status (0 or 1 vs. 2–4). Performance status is a measure of general health and ambulatory status. Two systems are used to measure it: the ECOG and the Karnofsky scale. See Appendix C.
4. Stage (I or II vs. III or IV).
5. Extranodal site involvement (0 or 1 vs. 2–4 sites).

People with two or more risk factors have a worse prognosis than those with no risk factors or with one. People with four or five risk factors have the worst prognosis. There was nothing Bob could do about his age, and he did have another risk factor, an elevated serum LDH level, which was abnormal on a repeat blood test, too.

Treatment Options

Treatment options and intensity of therapy depend on stage of disease, molecular signature and overall medical health, which for Bob is excellent for his age.

Surgery. Other than the biopsy, surgery is not part of Bob's treatment.

Chemotherapy. Combination chemotherapy is the key component of Bob's treatment. A number of drugs, usually three or four, are given on a 2–4 week cycle. CHOP chemotherapy consists of four drugs, cyclophosphamide (Cytoxan®), doxorubicin hydrochloride (Adriamycin®), vincristine (Oncovin®), and prednisone. Side effects include nausea and vomiting, and are reduced or prevented with drugs called anti-emetics; lowering of blood counts, which are carefully monitored and may require colony stimulating factors between cycles and some change in frequency of drug administration; heart damage, which can be monitored and likely avoided; and appetite and sleep disturbances, which can be helped somewhat with medicine and diet. This regimen has been in use for a few decades, so doctors have much experience with it.

A new monoclonal antibody treatment, rituximab (Rituxan®), is used in many instances in which tumor cells have CD-20 on the surface, as Bob's do. Because of Bob's molecular profiling and IPI risk, Bob and his doctor decided that rituximab will be added to his treatment, as part of a clinical trial to see if adding rituximab to CHOP will improve prognosis, as determined by patients' molecular profiles. (A molecular profile is a study of a tumor's genes and proteins using DNA microarray. See Appendix A.) This combined treatment is called CHOP-R. Bob and Holly read the consent form for the clinical trial and signed it after further discussion with the doctor.

Radiation therapy. A number of studies have shown that fewer cycles of chemotherapy, usually three to four, plus local (*involved field*) radiation of the tumor site can do as well as or better than more prolonged chemotherapy of six or more cycles. Other studies are still ongoing that compare different regimens with one another, and compare chemotherapy plus monoclonal antibody alone with combined radiation and the same chemotherapy-monoclonal antibody regimen. For Bob, the doctor plans to use CHOP-R, restage after two and possibly three cycles, and then change to radiation after the third or possibly fourth cycle, while continuing the rituximab, as on the clinical protocol, during the radiation. The radiation will be to the area of the stomach and will require twenty treatments, once a day for 5 days per week for 4 weeks. Each treatment will take less than an hour. Side effects are nausea, treated with anti-emetics, and possibly low blood counts.

Combination therapy. The use of both systemic therapy and radiation is called combination therapy or combined modality therapy. After two cycles of CHOP-R, the physician will use CT and PET scans to restage Bob's tumor, and if the tumor has shrunk, will go on to radiation therapy after the third cycle of CHOP-R. A fourth cycle may be used if the response to chemotherapy, as shown on PET and CT scans, is not complete.

In the course of their discussion with the doctors, Bob's wife Holly went on the Internet and looked up "stomach lymphoma." She asked the doctor about treatment with just antibiotics and maybe just a small dose of radiation. As the doctor explained, Holly had found information about a non-Hodgkin's lymphoma called a *MALT* (*mucosa associated lymphatic tissue*), also called *marginal zone lymphoma*. This is a low-grade lymphoma associated with a bacterial infection with H. pylori. The pathologist looked at the biopsy specimen for this and did not find it. The pathologist also performed immunohistochemistry studies that showed that Bob had diffuse large cell, B-cell lymphoma and not a MALT lymphoma. That was why the oncologist had believed it was so important to get the diagnosis right, even requiring a second biopsy, because treatments for the two lymphomas are so different. The doctor explained that molecular profiling (DNA microarray) of tumors is cutting-edge clinical science and that Bob may want to join a clinical trial that looks at treatment outcome based on molecular profiling as well as on the other features like the pathology of the tumor and Bob's risk factors according to the IPI.

Clinical trial. Bob and his wife decide that he should enter the clinical trial, which is sponsored by the cancer center where the pathologist worked who helped in the diagnosis. Bob has already undergone the biopsy needed for the molecular profiling. He visits the oncologists at the cancer center who will work with his oncologist on the treatment regimen and follow-up. Bob signs the informed consent document and is ready to go.

Personal Considerations

Bob has had few sick days in his life and is intent on working as much as possible. He has many sick days banked if he needs them. He plans to take off the day of chemotherapy and the day after, if necessary. He plans to have his radiation treatment in the mid-afternoon, so he can go to work first and then go home after treatment and take a nap before dinner.

Patient's Checklist

Name: Bob G.

Diagnosis

Type of tumor and tumor site: Non-Hodgkin's lymphoma—diffuse, B-cell type. CD-20 positive. Stomach.

Molecular profile: BCL-2 positive, other genes studied.

Clinical Staging Studies

Clinical stage: CS IEA

Blood tests: Normal except for LDH elevated at 2 times normal.

Imaging studies: CT scan—thickened stomach, about 25% involvement; nodes a little big but probably okay. PET scan—abnormal in stomach area only.

Pathological Staging Studies

Pathological stage: PS IEA

Additional biopsies: Repeat biopsy showed same type of lymphoma—read by special lymphoma expert at Major Cancer Center. Bone marrow—a few extra lymphocytes, but not lymphoma.

Treatment Options

Surgery

Not necessary other than for biopsy or if there is a perforation in stomach during treatment. That is not likely.

Radiation therapy

Used to be used as primary therapy for this type of lymphoma but is now part of combination therapy.

Region of body to be treated: Radiation will be to the upper stomach.

Duration of treatment: Will begin after 3 cycles of chemotherapy, assuming that the disease is going away. Radiation will take 4 weeks,

5 days per week. The treatment will take about an hour, including changing, getting the treatment, and seeing the doctor periodically.

Side effects: Some nausea and weight loss. Special diet supplements should be considered. Also, may want to schedule radiation for the mid-afternoon and take a few hours of sick leave each day. May drop my blood counts but doctor will follow that each week or more.

Systemic therapy

Drugs or agents to be used or considered: Combined chemotherapy with drugs called CHOP-R (cyclophosphamide, doxorubicin hydrochloride, vincristine and prednisone plus a monoclonal antibody called rituximab). Other regimens are available, including one called EPOCH.

Treatment schedule: Every 3 weeks for 9 weeks. A longer interval may be needed if blood counts do not recover quickly enough.

Side effects: Nausea and vomiting, which will be treated with anti-emetics; temporary hair loss; change in appetite from prednisone. Also sleeplessness. Low blood counts can be a problem, and doctors may need to use a drug called colony stimulating factor to raise white cell count. Rituxan® can cause flu-like symptoms. Watch for allergic reaction.

Heart damage is possible from doxorubicin hydrochloride (Adriamycin®) if many cycles are needed (more than 5 or 6), but doctors will monitor my heart.

Combination therapy

Plan is to start with 2 cycles of CHOP-R and check response with CT and PET scans.

Third cycle will be given followed by radiation therapy. Fourth cycle may be needed if tumor response is slow. If tumor doesn't go away, salvage chemotherapy would be needed. No need to discuss this now, as it is not likely to be needed.

Clinical trial

Clinical trial is available that looks at molecular profiling (DNA microarray) and how it relates to response to treatment. Will join this.

Throughout the trial I can be treated by my own oncologist, using the cancer center's protocol and visiting the center from time to time.

Summary of Treatment Options

Surgery not needed. Chemotherapy plus Rituxan® (CHOP-R) followed by restaging, followed by radiation or more chemotherapy before radiation.

This combination treatment regimen likely brings cure to about 80–90%.

Final Plan

CHOP-R times 2 cycles. Restage with CT and PET scan. If tumor has shrunk, proceed to third cycle of CHOP-R and then to radiation to stomach for 4 weeks, continuing Rituxan®.

Monthly follow up for 6 months, every 3–4 months after that until 2 years, then twice a year until 5 years, and yearly thereafter.

Bob's blended family has come to his support and are planning a 2-week-long victory trip to Europe after all the treatment is done and Bob feels better. Being a careful accountant, Bob also checks to see that his will and health directives are up to date. He hopes that his stomach will feel a bit better once he recovers from the treatment. He will continue using antacids until after the cancer treatment is done.

Final Plan

Bob has undergone careful clinical, pathological, and molecular staging for his non-Hodgkin's lymphoma. He will undergo therapy involving a limited number of cycles of CHOP-R on a clinical protocol and, if restaging is okay as expected, he will finish three cycles of chemotherapy and then a month of radiation. This will take about 4 months overall. Bob will need long-term follow-up with his medical and radiation oncologists and frequent follow-up with his internist. He has organized his time and life to eliminate as much stress as he can while continuing his work, which is very important to him. He and his wife look forward to a major family trip about 6 months from now and have begun planning that, too.

Case Study 2

Jane S.'s story illustrates the treatment options available for a person with a primary tumor in the breast. It describes all three standard treatments available to patients with the disease: surgery, radiation therapy, and systemic therapy. The type of information a patient with breast cancer would gather has been entered in Jane's Patient Checklist.

Medical History

Jane S., a healthy 47-year-old married woman, noticed a small irregularity in her right breast during a self-examination and consulted her family doctor. During a physical examination, he found a small lump about 1 inch in diameter on the outer half of her right breast. Although most lumps are not cancer, a person with a lump like Jane's needs to undergo a biopsy procedure. If the results of the biopsy are positive, the oncologist will discuss the treatment options with the woman and her family members.

Diagnosis

Jane's doctor referred her to a diagnostic radiologist for a mammogram, which revealed a small, solid (calcified) area that looked suspicious. The radiologist identified the specific area involved using a procedure called a *needle localization,* in which the radiologist places the tip of a needle into the abnormal area. Because many abnormalities found on mammography are too small to detect by touch, the needle localization performed by the radiologist allows the surgeon to find the lesion. The surgeon then performs a lumpectomy by removing the lump and some normal tissue around it which the radiologist has identified. A pathologist subsequently takes mammographic x-rays of the specimen to ensure that all the calcifications have been removed.

Patient's Checklist

Name: Jane S.

Diagnosis

Type of tumor and tumor site: Adenocarcinoma of the breast.

Clinical Staging Studies

Clinical stage: CS IIA (T2N0M0). Tumor measuring 2.5 centimeters completely removed. Margins are clear. Test for estrogen receptors was positive.

Gene expression profiling done: Tissue analysis for HER2/neu was negative.

Blood tests: All normal.

Imaging studies: Mammogram before the biopsy showed a small area of calcification. After the biopsy, a second mammogram showed that all the calcification was removed. Chest x-ray and bone scan were normal.

Pathological Staging Studies

Pathological stage: PS IIB (T2N1M0).

Additional biopsies: In sample of eight lymph nodes, one was involved with the tumor. CS changed to PS because of positive nodes.

Treatment Options

Surgery

Extent of procedure and length of hospitalization: Mastectomy requires 1–2 days in hospital. Lumpectomy can be performed on an outpatient basis. Surgery for pathological staging of lymph nodes is an outpatient procedure.

Side effects: Minor discomfort and swelling from node sampling.

Expected results: Mastectomy produces same results as lumpectomy plus radiation.

Radiation therapy

Region of body to be treated: Breast and chest wall.

Duration of treatment: 6.5 weeks, 5 days per week.

Side effects: Short term—skin redness; long term—less than 1% chance of lung injury and 1%–2% chance of swelling of arm.

Expected results: Same as with modified radical mastectomy. Ten-year survival is approximately 60%–70%.

Systemic therapy

Drugs or agents to be used or considered: Doxorubicin, cyclophosphamide and one of the taxol drugs—docetaxel or paclitaxel—depending on the treatment arm of the study. Gemcitabine is also a possibility. Toxicity information sheet will be provided by the research team.

Hormonal therapy will begin after the chemotherapy.

Side effects: Short term—nausea, hair loss, lowered blood counts and small risk of infection. Long term—loss of menstrual function and onset of hot flashes.

Combination therapy

Chemotherapy for about 5 months, followed by radiation for about 6.5 weeks (for a total of about 6 or 7 months), followed by hormonal therapy. The exact timing will depend on the arm of the clinical trial protocol.

Clinical trial

NASBP B-38 study. More detailed information will be provided on side effect and specifics of schedule.

Summary of Treatment Options

Mastectomy or breast conserving treatment.

For breast conserving treatment, partial breast irradiation or whole breast irradiation.

Chemotherapy—will use clinical research protocol.

Final Plan

Biopsy with tissue sent for special studies including molecular analysis.

Lymph node dissection.

NSABP B-38 trial with chemotherapy, then radiation therapy, for a total of about 6 or 7 months, followed by longer-term hormonal therapy.

Staging Studies

Clinical staging. A few days after the surgical procedure, another mammogram of Jane's breast confirmed that the calcifications had been completely removed. The tumor mass measured 2.5 centimeters in diameter (approximately 1 inch) and contained invasive cancer (adenocarcinoma). Routine blood tests, a chest x-ray, and a bone scan all proved to be normal.

The pathologist cut thin sections of the removed breast tissue, examined them under the microscope, and found no traces of cancer at the margins of the tumor. The diagnosis of invasive breast cancer was made, and, according to the TNM staging system, the tumor was classified as CS T2N0M0 because its diameter was between 2 and 5 centimeters, no lymph nodes appeared to be involved, and the disease had not metastasized.

When tumor tissue was sent to a laboratory for special studies, the test for estrogen receptors was positive—the cancer cells had estrogen receptors on their surface. This information was useful because tumor cells with estrogen receptors on their surface are more likely to respond to antiestrogen therapy than are cells that lack these receptors. The pathologist also examined the tissue to identify some of the tumor's molecular and cellular properties. The pathologist stained the tissue for the protein HER2/ neu, which was negative. A sample was sent off for gene expression profiling, although the oncologist and patient realized that this is a new technology without a definitely proven track record. They felt that it might help in decision making for adjuvant therapy and possibly other uses down the line; however, they would use the lymph node status as the primary test for determining the need for chemotherapy or hormonal therapy.

Pathological staging. In Jane's case, pathological staging was not completed at this point. Instead, an overall plan involving some form of combination therapy was developed for her care.

Treatment Options

Surgery. Two surgical options are available to treat localized breast cancer. One option is a modified radical mastectomy, during which the surgeon removes the entire breast, some of the tissue underlying the breast, and the lymph nodes in the patient's axilla (armpit). Following removal of the breast, breast reconstruction can be performed if the patient wishes. In some cases, certain microscopic features of a tumor make a mastectomy preferable to radiation therapy. In other cases, certain pathological features, such as a tumor that involves the chest wall or skin, make it necessary to use radiation therapy after the mastectomy.

The other surgical option is a lumpectomy, which has already been done in Jane's case. A lumpectomy is followed by radiation therapy. Although a patient's lymph nodes may feel normal, about one-third of patients have cancer in some of the nodes. The presence of cancer in the lymph nodes is an important factor in determining whether a patient needs adjuvant chemotherapy after the radiation therapy. If Jane elects to have a mastectomy, the nodes will be biopsied during the procedure. If Jane decides not to have a mastectomy, her lymph nodes will be sampled in a separate surgical procedure on an outpatient basis before radiation therapy begins. She ultimately chooses to have the sampling procedure. Jane considered having the lymph nodes sampled first using a sentinel node biopsy, but she decided to go ahead with the regular axillary dissection.

Radiation. The radiation therapy is administered 5 days a week for 6 or 7 weeks to the normal breast and the chest wall. Depending on the presence and number of affected lymph nodes, the nodes might or might not be included in the field of radiation. The major side effect of the treatment is redness of the skin in the field of radiation. This reaction is usually mild and subsides within a few weeks after the treatment ends. The possible late effects include a less than 1 percent chance of injury to the lungs and a 1 or 2 percent risk of swelling of the arm. The rate of 10-year overall survival is 60 to 70 percent.

Jane asked her radiation oncologists about a new treatment option someone in her breast cancer support group told her about called partial breast irradiation, or PBI. The doctor told Jane that there are a number of ways of doing PBI, but that this is a relatively new procedure and despite the wide publicity, there is only a limited amount of long-term information available about it. Jane's radiation oncologist participates in a cooperative group trial, Radiation Therapy Oncology Group, RTOG 0413, that is a multigroup study. Although Jane is eligible, because Jane has a T2 and N1 tumor her doctor prefers to use the more standard treatment and believes that this is a more conservative approach. When Jane has a meeting with the medical oncologist and radiation oncologist to discuss the overall plan for her treatment, they decide to use another clinical trial for chemotherapy and therefore think it best to stick with the more standard whole breast method of irradiation.

Systemic therapy. That adjuvant therapy provides benefit in terms of reduced recurrence and improved survival for many subsets of patients made this a complex decision for Jane. There are many factors to consider in understanding the precise benefit of this therapy, including clinical and molecular features. Because Jane has lymph node–involved breast cancer with positive estrogen receptors, she will undergo systemic chemotherapy plus hormonal therapy. She has looked over many of the breast cancer sites on the Internet, including medical articles she located using the National Library of Medicine Web site. Her new friends in the breast cancer support group help. However, given the wide range of regimens, Jane remains uncertain of which is the best choice. She concludes that there is no one single best choice but rather a number of appropriate treatment options.

Jane's doctor agrees with her and explains that most experts recommend chemotherapy plus hormonal therapy for premenopausal women who have breast cancer with an involved node, but

B-38 SCHEMA

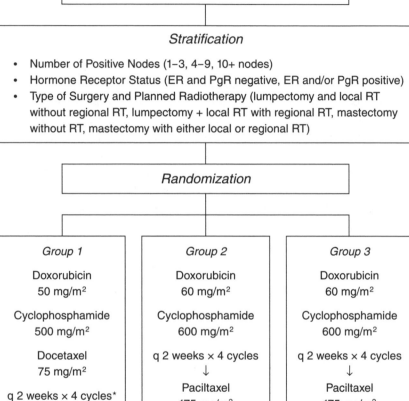

Operable Breast Cancer
Histologically Positive Nodes

Stratification

- Number of Positive Nodes (1–3, 4–9, 10+ nodes)
- Hormone Receptor Status (ER and PgR negative, ER and/or PgR positive)
- Type of Surgery and Planned Radiotherapy (lumpectomy and local RT without regional RT, lumpectomy + local RT with regional RT, mastectomy without RT, mastectomy with either local or regional RT)

Randomization

Group 1

Doxorubicin
50 mg/m²

Cyclophosphamide
500 mg/m²

Docetaxel
75 mg/m²

q 2 weeks × 4 cycles*
↓
Hormonal therapy**

Group 2

Doxorubicin
60 mg/m²

Cyclophosphamide
600 mg/m²

q 2 weeks × 4 cycles
↓
Paciltaxel
175 mg/m²

q 2 weeks × 4 cycles*
↓
Hormonal Therapy**

Group 3

Doxorubicin
60 mg/m²

Cyclophosphamide
600 mg/m²

q 2 weeks × 4 cycles
↓
Paciltaxel
175 mg/m²

Gemcitabine
2000 mg/m²

q 2 weeks × 4 cycles*
↓
Hormonal Therapy**

* Primary prophylaxis with pegfilgrastim or filgrastim is required. See Section 8.0 for details.
** Women with ER-positive and/or PgR-positive tumors will begin hormonal therapy no sooner than 3 weeks and no later than 12 weeks following the last dose of chemotherapy. Protocol requirements for hormonal therapy are outlined in Section 8.4.

there are still choices between regimens involving different schedules and drugs. Jane and her doctor decide that the best way to get to a decision would be to join in a clinical trial, which would help her and also help generate new knowledge. Jane's medical oncologist participates in clinical trials by the National Surgical Adjuvant Breast Project (NSABP), so they choose an NSABP B-38 trial. The schema of this clinical trial is shown in figure 9.1. Jane discusses the protocol with her doctor and the research nurse and signs the informed consent.

Combination therapy. The clinical study protocol determines the parameters for the combination therapy. The sequence of treatments will depend on which arm of the study is selected by the randomization procedure. Having had the detailed discussions about all the options, Jane is very happy to learn that all aspects of her treatment on the clinical trial are based on formal guidelines and that there is careful quality assurance so that the pathology is reviewed and the drugs and radiation are given according to protocol.

Clinical trial. The NSABP trial will be followed.

Personal Considerations

Jane has a number of personal matters to consider while deciding which course of treatment to choose. A modified radical mastectomy can have a serious impact on a woman's body image, and chemotherapy means that she will lose her hair. Female members of Jane's family will have concerns about their own health, and Jane will probably want to talk with her oncologists and a genetic counselor about a screening program for family members. As I mentioned in Chapter 2, however, a genetic susceptibility

---

Fig. 9.1. A representative schema for a clinical trial (opposite)

Jane will be treated in the NSABP B-38 trial. She is eligible because she has operable breast cancer with histologically positive nodes (top box). Before randomization to treatment she will be assigned a category according to the criteria listed in the second box (stratification). Then the NSABP statistical center will let her doctor know which group Jane has been randomly assigned to for treatment (lower boxes).

to cancer involves the potential for problems regarding insurance coverage and job discrimination as well as the obvious medical and psychological issues. Therefore, it is necessary to talk with a counselor before testing is done for a hereditary predisposition.

An immediate practical concern Jane faces is the time required for combination therapy. Jane must ensure that her children are cared for properly. On days when Jane receives treatment, her husband or a friend will take over the car pool rounds for Jane's 10-year-old daughter and her friends who attend music lessons. Because Jane plans to continue working during her treatments, she will need to schedule her radiotherapy appointments near the end of the workday. Thus, she will have to arrange to leave work a little early, and she may have to take a day off when she receives chemotherapy.

Final Plan

Jane decides against having a mastectomy and instead opts for breast-conserving treatment. In a separate surgical procedure the surgeon removes eight lymph nodes from her right armpit, and the pathologist discovers that one node is involved with the tumor. The clinical stage of her disease changes from CS IIA to PS IIB (T2N1M0). Jane will participate in the clinical trial. She has developed a good working relationship with the oncology research nurse who will help keep Jane up to date on the protocol schedule. Jane is assured that the protocol has flexibility to account for specific problems that may arise such as low blood counts, infection, or other reactions. So, the protocol has strict quality assurance and also very clear guidelines for necessary schedule changes to accommodate what actually happens to each patient.

Jane is very optimistic about the chance for a full recovery. She is grateful for all the progress in treatment resulting from many decades of clinical and laboratory research and for the willingness of so many people before her to participate in clinical trials. She is happy to participate in a randomized trial as it will give her good treatment and also help others in the future.

After a brief discussion with a genetic counselor, Jane decides against genetic testing because she has no family history of breast or ovarian cancer. She was happy to have the molecular profile study of her breast tumor done, although it did not affect her decision making. She learned from her breast cancer support group that many insurance plans do not yet pay for this test, and she understands that it takes time for new technology to undergo the appropriate standardization, FDA approval, and validation by additional clinical trials. She knows that premature or inappropriate use of new technology could create harm. She tells her oncologist that if a researcher wants to use her tumor profile data in a study, she would be happy to provide the information. Finally, with the help of her new friends in the support group, she decides to be an active campaigner for increased support for cancer research and an advocate for clinical trials.

Case Study 3

In this case study we see how a person might deal with a cancer that is discovered during a routine blood test, as well as how a person who is diagnosed with an early stage cancer might choose between two effective treatments for such a cancer. Prostate cancer discovered not by either a physical examination or imaging studies but by the PSA blood test—as Jim K.'s cancer was discovered—is sometimes called *incidental*. The PSA test is a test that is used routinely by many physicians to screen older men for prostate cancer. The clinical and pathological features of the individual prostate cancer determine whether the cancer requires immediate treatment or not. As the PSA test detects more and more prostate cancers in older men, it has become crucial to answer the question of who needs immediate treatment and who can be observed and be treated only if the disease progresses; this approach is called watchful waiting. This question is relevant both to individual patients, who experience the side effects of treatment, and to those who decide on health policy, because the treatment of so many men can be expensive. Thus, it must be shown that there are real benefits of screening and early treatment—and that men are not being unnecessarily alarmed about and treated for a condition that is unlikely to affect their health. Jim K.'s Patient Checklist indicates the kind of information which would be included for a man with incidental prostate cancer.

Medical History

Jim K. is a healthy 68-year-old married, retired man who is an avid skier and hiker. Although his sexual functioning has declined in recent years, he is still sexually active. A routine physical examination, including a rectal examination, indicated that his prostate was normal. However, the result of his PSA test was slightly elevated—4.5, versus a normal value of less than 4. Though it was very slow, the rise in Jim's PSA concerned his doctor. On Jim's PSA tests over the last 7 years, the numbers were 2.5, 2.2, 2.7, 2.6, 2.5, 3.6, and 4.5. This represented an increase in PSA velocity with a doubling time of a little more than 2 years (going from 2.5 to 4.5 over the last 2 years). The results of all the other blood chemistry tests and his blood count were normal.

Jim had heard about many of his friends and public figures who were diagnosed with prostate cancer, so he agreed to have a sonogram through the rectum (*transrectal ultrasound;* TRUS) and a biopsy of the prostate, in which a biopsy needle is used to remove three cores of tissue from each side of the gland, called a sextant biopsy.

Diagnosis

The sonogram did not reveal any abnormalities. However, the needle biopsy revealed that one of the three cores on the left side of the gland contained cancer cells (Gleason score, 6 out of 10) and 20 percent of that core was cancerous. The right side of the gland was benign.

Staging Studies

Clinical staging. As the doctor expected, a bone scan and a pelvic CT scan were normal. An MRI performed using a special coil placed in the rectum (endorectal MRI) showed an abnormality in the left side of the gland that did not reach the capsule. According to the TNM system, the stage of Jim's cancer was CS T1CNOMO, meaning that no mass could be felt, the tumor was

Patient's Checklist

Name: Jim K.

Diagnosis

Type of tumor and tumor site: "Incidental" cancer of the prostate which is localized in the gland.

Clinical Staging Studies

Clinical stage: CS A1 or TIC.

Blood tests: Prostate specific antigen (PSA) test of 4.5 (normal result is less than 4). PSA doubling time greater than 2 years. All other chemistry tests, and blood count are normal.

Imaging studies: Bone scan, CT scan of the pelvis, and transrectal ultrasound of the prostate (sonogram) all normal. Endorectal MR showed abnormality <1/4 of gland and confined to gland.

Pathological Staging Studies

Pathological stage: Initial biopsy had Gleason score of 6/10 in one of three biopsy cores on the left side of the gland; 20% of this core contained cancer. On the right side of the gland, all three biopsy cores were normal.

Additional biopsies: No additional biopsies were performed.

Treatment Options

Careful observation with no immediate treatment.

Surgery

Extent of procedure and length of hospitalization: Nerve-sparing radical prostatectomy, which requires less than 1 week in hospital, about 2–3 weeks with a catheter, and 4–6 weeks recuperation at home.

Side effects: Short term—loss of urinary control for few weeks or months, loss of ability to have sexual relations, which can last many months. Long term—40%–70% chance of permanent loss of sexual potency, helped with drugs treating erectile dysfunction; 2% chance of permanent urinary incontinence.

Expected results: Approximately 80% overall survival at 10 years. If the pathological exam shows a higher Gleason score, more extensive involvement of prostate by tumor, or cancer cells beyond the capsule, the prognosis may fall to only 60% survival at 15 years.

*Radiation therapy

Region of body to be treated: Prostate and surrounding margin.

External beam. 3D-conformal radiation or intensity modulated radiation therapy (IMRT).

Duration of treatment: 38 treatments, 5 days per week for almost 8 weeks.

Side effects: Short term—urinary frequency and bowel urgency, which usually clear up within 1–3 months after radiation. Long term—10% chance of blood occasionally in urine or stools, 2%–5% chance of bothersome bowel or urinary problems, 50%–70% chance of inability to have sexual relations.

Brachytherapy. There are 2 forms of brachytherapy, high dose rate temporary implant or permanent implant with radioactive seeds. These use radioactive seeds made of either iodine or palladium.

Duration of treatment: Implanting the seeds requires one procedure lasting a few hours.

Side effects: Short-term—In the first few weeks there can be urinary frequency and a risk of urinary obstruction. Long term—2–5% risk of urinary discomfort. Impotence, inability to have sexual relations—40–50%. Helped with drugs treating erectile dysfunction.

Expected results: Disease-free survival is 90% at 5 years, 75% at 10 years.

*Systemic therapy

Drugs or agents to be used or considered: None.

*Combination therapy

None planned.

Summary of Treatment Options

Observation. No treatment unless disease progresses.

Nerve-sparing radical prostatectomy.

Radiation therapy using external beam radiation therapy with 3D-conformal radiation or intensity modulate radiation therapy. Brachytherapy with radioactive seeds or high dose rate brachytherapy.

Final Plan

Radiation therapy with brachytherapy.

---

detected only with a routine blood test, the CT scan detected no evidence that lymph nodes were involved, and the bone scan was normal. "T1C" is a relatively new designation, indicating that the tumor was detected with a routine blood test. In Jim's case, the tumor was confined to less than one-quarter of the gland and the Gleason score was low, so his prognosis was excellent. Other men with T1C cancers may have different pathological features that would predict a poorer prognosis.

Pathological staging. No additional biopsies were done.

Treatment Options

Before discussing Jim's treatment options, an important question to ask is whether his cancer will ever become a clinical problem. The answer will depend on the issues discussed in Chapters 3 and 6: the natural history of the tumor (how it will behave if it is not treated), the person's overall medical condition, and his expected life span. All treatments for prostate cancer have side effects. Will treatment cause more problems for Jim than it solves?

Because Jim is a healthy, active 68-year-old and has a good chance of living another 15 to 20 years, he prefers to deal with his medical problem sooner rather than later. He is concerned about maintaining his sexual potency, but he would worry more about an untreated cancer and is willing to accept this side effect if he will be able to maintain his other activities. Consequently, he believes that treatment is the logical choice.

The fact that Jim's disease is localized to the prostate gland and has good pathological features means that he doesn't need systemic treatment. For prostate cancer, systemic treatment involves removing testosterone (a male hormone) by using drugs. Jim's two choices are local modalities: surgery or radiation therapy. No clinical trials have adequately compared the effectiveness of the two treatments. In practice, however, the survival rates for both treatments appear to be similar, so the choice of treatment would primarily depend on the different side effects.

Surgery. If Jim and his doctor choose surgery, the procedure will be a nerve-sparing radical prostatectomy, which requires one week of hospitalization. In this procedure, the urologist attempts to remove the entire prostate gland while sparing the nerves on one or both sides of the gland which control erections. The patient's bladder is catheterized for 2 or 3 weeks, and the patient will need to recuperate at home for 4 to 6 weeks. The chance that the tumor will be removed completely is approximately 90 percent. With careful follow-up using PSA tests, the patient's chances of overall survival 10 years after surgery are approximately 80 percent. After the prostate is removed, a pathologist will examine the entire gland carefully. If she finds features that indicate more extensive tumor involvement of the gland or spread of the tumor beyond the capsule, or if she finds that the patient's Gleason grade is higher than the original score, then his prognosis would be poorer. If disease is spread locally beyond the gland, postoperative radiation therapy may be recommended.

The short-term side effects of surgery include loss of urinary control (incontinence), which can last a few weeks or months or even longer, and loss of sexual potency, which can either last many months or be permanent. The long-term effects include a 50 to 70 percent risk of permanent impotence and a 2 percent risk of permanent urinary incontinence. Impotence can be treated with drugs for treating erectile dysfunction, which are sometimes effective.

Radiation therapy. If Jim and his doctor choose external beam radiation therapy, his prostate gland and local lymph nodes will be irradiated 5 days per week for 7 or 8 weeks for a total of 38 treatments. For as long as 3 months during and after treatment, he will experience frequent urination and bowel movements. In the long term, he will have a 10 percent chance that blood would occasionally appear in his urine or stools, a 2 to 5 percent chance of having troublesome urinary or bowel problems, and a 50 to 70 percent chance of permanent impotence, which may be successfully treated with drugs for treating erectile dysfunction. Disease-free survival rates for men with this stage of prostate cancer after radiation therapy are about 75 percent at 10 years. An alternative form of radiation is a radioactive implant (brachytherapy), which has become increasingly popular for patients with a favorable prognosis, like Jim. High risk factors that would affect outcome and treatment selection may be different in different staging systems, but examples of high risk factors include PSA above 10 ng/ml, big prostate nodule greater than half of one lobe (T2B), or Gleason score of 7 or higher. The presence of one risk factor means the patient is intermediate risk, and two or three of them means the patient is high risk. The high-risk group will have hormonal therapy as part of the treatment. That therapy may also be used for some intermediate risk patients, but not the low-risk group. Also, for deciding between brachytherapy and external beam radiation the local anatomy is important; if the nodule is at the back edge of the gland, it is hard to get enough of the seeds around the tumor. Seed brachytherapy involves a one-day procedure during which the radioactive seeds are placed in the prostate gland. Side effects include mild discomfort with urination for a few weeks and possible temporary urinary obstruction. Impotence occurs in less than half of patients and can be treated with drugs for treating erectile dysfunction.

Systemic or combination therapy. Jim doesn't need either form of treatment.

Clinical trial. In some clinical trials, researchers are comparing the effectiveness of the standard dosage of radiation and higher dosages. Higher dosages can kill more cancer cells but also can cause more damage to normal tissue. The higher doses are usually for the cancers with less favorable prognoses (high and intermediate risk, as described above).

Personal Considerations

Jim has always been physically active, and the potential side effects of surgery and radiation therapy are important to him. After surgery, he would be unable to engage in very strenuous activity for about 6 months. An even longer-term problem might be an inability to control his urination when he exerts himself. After external beam irradiation, he might find that because the treatment has scarred parts of his bladder and rectum, he would urinate or defecate more often. Brachytherapy seemed to have fewer rectal side effects. The new class of drugs for treating erectile dysfunction are helping many men obtain at least a partial erection after all forms of local prostate cancer therapy. Jim and his wife both think that a chance of urinary incontinence would really affect Jim's lifestyle. They are encouraged by all the new research on developing better treatments, and they realize that even if this treatment doesn't cure him, there is good second line treatment. Jim has many years to go and it is not likely he will die from prostate cancer. They conclude that brachytherapy is a good choice.

Final Plan

Jim understands that he is likely to do well with either surgery or radiation therapy. But because he is so physically active, he decides that the risk of incontinence with surgery, although extremely low, is not a risk he is willing to take. Therefore, he decides on radiation therapy with brachytherapy.

Case Study 4

This case study involving Mary B. illustrates a situation in which long-term survival is rare. In such a case the purpose of treatment is usually palliative rather than curative: that is, the treatment is given to alleviate the patient's symptoms, not to cure the disease. The kind of information about diagnosis, treatment options, and so forth which would be needed in such a case has been recorded in the Patient's Checklist for Mary.

Medical History

Mary B., a 57-year-old accountant, had been suffering increasingly from headaches for several months. She is divorced, has two married sons, and shares her home with her mother, who, at 79 years old, is still active and self-sufficient. Mary's doctor ordered a CT scan of her brain, which revealed a tumor.

Diagnosis

Mary was referred to a neurosurgeon, who ordered an MRI scan to better define the site and boundaries of the tumor. The surgeon then performed a biopsy. During surgery, the neurosurgeon found that he could remove only a limited amount of the tumor without damaging Mary's ability to function. The tissue that was removed revealed a glioblastoma, an extremely malignant tumor.

Staging Studies

Because the MRI defined the extent of Mary's tumor, no additional clinical or pathological tests were required.

Treatment Options

Because Mary's prognosis is poor, no effective standard treatment is available. However, if she decides to pursue standard treatment, most doctors would choose radiation therapy and chemotherapy. Because cure rates for Mary's disease are extremely low, these treatments would be palliative (they would ease her symptoms) rather than offer the possibility of cure.

Surgery. The biopsy and removal of some of the tumor was the only surgery possible. If she was not already seen at a major medical center, Mary might choose to go there, or at least to send her MR films to them to see if they could possibly remove more of the tumor.

Patient's Checklist

Name: Mary B.

Diagnosis

Type of tumor and tumor site: Brain tumor: glioblastoma multiforme.

Clinical Staging Studies

No staging system used.

Blood tests: No specific tests.

Imaging studies: CT and MRI scans of the brain revealed the tumor.

Pathological Staging Studies

None.

Treatment Options

Surgery

Extent of procedure and length of hospitalization: Removal of as much of the tumor as possible without causing loss of function. Requires 4–5 days in hospital.

Side effects: Hair loss from shaving of surgical site. Possibly some loss of neurological function, depending on the site of the tumor.

Expected results: Median survival of 6 months with surgery alone.

Radiation therapy

Region of the body to be treated: Tumor and surrounding brain (margins).

Duration of treatment: 5 treatments per week for 6 weeks.

Side effects: Short term—hair loss, skin irritation. Long term—possible brain injury, depending on dosage used.

Expected results: Will increase median survival time by approximately 4 additional months (to 10 months).

Systemic therapy

Drugs or agents to be used: temozolomide.

Treatment schedule: Oral, daily with radiation. Then 6 cycles, each lasting 28 days with pills for the first 5 days.

Hospitalization required? No.

Side effects: Short term—nausea, low blood counts. Long term—probably none.

Expected results: Can add a few months to survival (median, 14 months).

Combination therapy

Surgery, followed by radiation therapy plus chemotherapy, then chemotherapy.

Expected results: The use of the three treatment modalities may increase survival to 12 or 14 months, perhaps longer.

Clinical trial

A Phase I or Phase II clinical trial that is developing a new treatment, which may consist of (1) new techniques of radiation therapy that increase the dose to the tumor, (2) new drugs (radiation sensitizers) that make radiation more effective, or (3) new molecular-targeted drugs or biological agents.

Summary of Treatment Options

Surgery followed by radiation therapy.

Surgery followed by radiation therapy, then chemotherapy.

Surgery followed by radiation therapy and chemotherapy used simultaneously.

Final Plan

Simultaneous radiation therapy plus chemotherapy, followed by chemotherapy after irradiation is completed. Clinical trial when disease gets worse.

Radiation. If Mary chooses to undergo radiation therapy, she would receive 5 treatments per week for 6 weeks to the tumor and the surrounding tissue. This treatment would be likely to increase her survival time by about 4 months. The short-term side effects would include hair loss and skin irritation. Depending on the dosage of radiation, Mary might experience additional damage to her brain over the longer term.

Systemic therapy. Since Mary is basically healthy, her physicians would use a drug called temozolomide (Temadar®) that is given by pill daily along with radiation and followed by 6 cycles of chemotherapy with pills for 5 days every 4 weeks. The major side effects are nausea, vomiting, and low blood counts.

Clinical trial. If Mary is interested in participating in a Phase I or Phase II clinical trial, she can find out what trials are available by consulting her doctor, a cancer center, or the National Cancer Institute. Some of these clinical trials are investigating new techniques of radiation therapy involving higher dosages or new drugs called radiation sensitizers, which increase the effectiveness of irradiation. Other trials are testing new anticancer drugs or biological agents such as gene therapy or molecular-targeted therapy.

Personal Considerations

For obvious reasons, Mary needs time to adjust to the shock of discovering that she has a fatal disease. She needs to make plans for someone to help her mother. Fortunately, her sister lives nearby, and one of her sons lives in the next town. Her doctor may alleviate some of her emotional pain by pointing out that many patients in her situation do reasonably well and enjoy a good quality of life for many months or even years. When Mary is ready to receive this information, she should be advised that handling her legal and financial affairs as soon as possible will help her and her relatives avoid frustration later.

Hospice programs have made a dramatic improvement in the quality of life for patients and families. With such a serious illness, Mary is likely to need hospice care at some time, a decision she will make with her doctors.

Final Plan

Mary will take the new combination of radiation plus temozolomide. She will definitely participate in a clinical trial at the time that her tumor gets worse (progresses). She hopes that the new treatment will not only benefit her but also provide new information that will benefit future patients.

Afterword

In my practice, I have found that patients and families were capable of making wise decisions once they had the tools available to make those decisions. Knowledgeable, well-informed patients are extremely valuable allies of the health care professional involved in cancer care, because such patients are able to participate actively and more comfortably in the entire process of cancer care — from the decision-making stage through the period of treatment to long-term follow-up.

My intention in writing this guidebook was to help you and members of your family feel more comfortable in dealing with your illness and, if you were faced with a choice of treatments, to give you the information you need to participate in making decisions about treatment. My wish is that all people with cancer can deal with the personal as well as the medical issues that inevitably arise when cancer is diagnosed. In the face of the devastating feelings that come with the diagnosis of cancer, many of my patients have altered their life objectives and priorities. They now live fuller and more meaningful lives than they did before the diagnosis. I feel extremely fortunate to have so many people with cancer teaching me about life and living.

This book would not have been possible without the assistance of Elizabeth Bowman, who helped to shape the first edition of the book, and my editor at the Johns Hopkins University Press, Jacqueline Wehmueller, whose wisdom and experience brought this effort to conclusion. I also thank my wife, Karolynn, and Davi and Bruce Chabner for their editorial advice, and Susan Lantz for editorial assistance on the second edition.

The advances made in cancer research have been dramatic since the first edition, and this new knowledge is affecting the outcome of cancer treatment, albeit much more slowly than we want. Obtaining time and money for research is always a challenge, and I am continuously impressed by the efforts of my colleagues, the research community, and the public figures who lend their support for this noble cause. The second edition of *Understanding Cancer* emphasizes clinical trials even more than the first edition, as there are now so many new treatments that need to be studied. My three decades as an oncologist have constantly taught me about human courage and determination, and I am sure I express on behalf of all of us engaged in the war on cancer our enormous gratitude for the altruism and courage of the people who volunteer to be in clinical trials.

Achieving success in cancer care is best done with the patient as an integral part of a partnership. I would welcome your feedback in writing regarding how useful you found this book to be, as well as your suggestions for improving it. You may write to me in care of

The Johns Hopkins University Press
2715 N. Charles Street
Baltimore, MD 21218-4363

Cancer Molecular Biology

In Chapter 2, fundamental concepts about the structure and function of normal cells and cancer cells are described. The major components of a cell are highlighted in figure 2.1, and figure 2.2 summarizes the stages in a cell division cycle, in which one cell divides into two cells. Molecular, cellular, and structural biologists have developed elegant methods for studying the fundamental processes within a cell. Some of these methods—the ones that are directly related to the etiology and diagnosis of cancer—are described here.

Studying Genes

Chromosomes are composed of genes. In the process described below, genes are the blueprint for making proteins, and it is these proteins by which genes actually function in the cell. Only part of the gene is made into proteins, whereas other parts are not. These other parts can be regulatory parts, by which the gene is controlled, or they can be "silent"—that is, without a currently known function (though over the past 5 years scientists have learned that the silent part of genes is active in controlling which genes are expressed). The parts of a gene which are made into protein are called *exons,* and the parts between the exons are called *introns.*

Gene Transcription

Gene transcription is the process during which messenger RNA (mRNA) is made out of a DNA molecule; through this process, genetic information is transferred from the DNA to the mRNA. Figure A.1 details the process of gene transcription. The region that controls each gene is situated before, or upstream of, the part of the gene which is transcribed. The messenger RNA (mRNA) made during gene transcription contains all the information needed to make new proteins. The mRNA is processed and transported into the cytoplasm, where, on structures called ribosomes, it is translated into a new protein.

For a gene to be activated, the proper proteins must be in place on the gene's control region. The regulatory proteins that activate gene transcription (again, transforming DNA into RNA) are called *transcription factors*. Other regulatory proteins can repress, or inactivate, gene transcription.

Whether a gene is transcribed will depend on signals from within or outside the cell. For example, as was described in Chapter 2, molecules called receptors on the surface of the cell can be activated by growth factors produced by other cells. These growth factors (or *ligands*) bind to the receptor and activate a process called *signal transduction*, which involves a communication network within the cell by which a receptor is activated and exerts control over the expression of a gene.

The process of gene transcription is carefully regulated by stimulatory and inhibitory processes that maintain a tight balance. In a cancer cell, any one of these processes can be abnormal: the growth factor, the growth-factor receptor, the signal transduction pathway, the regulatory proteins, the regulatory region of the gene itself, or the gene product. These different processes provide novel targets for cancer therapy.

The functions of RNA are much more complex than once thought. That is not entirely surprising, considering that life depended on RNA long before DNA came into existence. RNA can function as an enzyme, called a *ribozyme*. Very recently scientists have shown that small pieces of RNA can regulate genes and also

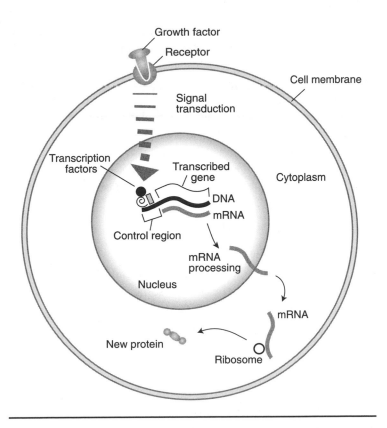

Fig. A.1. Some of the processes by which a gene is activated

The genes are composed of DNA, which is in the nucleus. Each gene has a control region that is situated before (upstream of) the part of the gene which is transcribed. During gene transcription, messenger RNA (mRNA) is produced; mRNA has all the information needed to make new proteins. The mRNA is processed and transported to the cytoplasm of the cell, where it is translated into a new protein on structures called ribosomes.

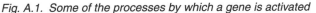

translation of mRNA into protein. By a process called RNA interference (RNAi) small pieces of RNA actually help turn genes on and off.

DNA exists in the cell in a very organized manner. The DNA is surrounded by proteins called *histones*. The histones are involved in silencing genes. Enzymes that change the histones (by processes called *methylation/demethylation* and *acetylation/deactylation*) can also determine which genes are on and off. These processes can affect many genes at one time. Because they change the function of genes but do not change the actual structure of the DNA bases, these processes of methylation and acetylation are called *epigenetic* modifiers. It is known that normal genes may be silenced in a cancer. This is another way, in addition to mutation or loss of a gene, that gene function can be altered. There are already drugs in clinical use that affect methylation and acetylation.

Studying Genes in the Laboratory
Karyotype Analysis

Some abnormalities in the genes of a cell can be seen under the microscope by looking at the chromosomes. To examine the chromosomes, scientists first must make the cell divide; then all 23 pairs of chromosomes are stained and analyzed. This process is called a *karyotype analysis.* In a karyotype analysis large abnormalities that occur in the structure of the chromosome can be seen. Figure A.2 illustrates three possible abnormalities.

The chromosomes shown in the first part (1.) of figure A.2 are normal: there are only two chromosomes, and both have the normal amount of DNA (neither of them is missing material or has additional material that doesn't belong to it). One of the chromosomes is from Parent A, the other from Parent B.

In the first abnormality (2.) shown in figure A.2, there are three chromosomes: two from Parent A and one from Parent B. This situation is called a *trisomy.* If the trisomy occurs on chromosome 21, the child will be born with Down's syndrome.

In the second abnormal situation (3.) in figure A.2, there is a *deletion* on one of the chromosomes — that is, part of the chromosome is missing. This may be important, because the genes that were located in the missing piece of DNA may be vital to the function of the cell. In this case, the loss of the gene produces an abnormal cell.

The third abnormality (4.) is a chromosome that has suffered

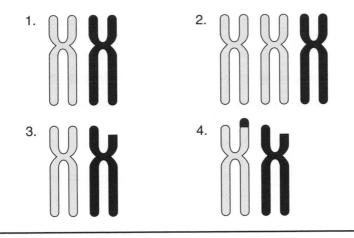

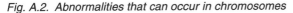

Fig. A.2. *Abnormalities that can occur in chromosomes*

These are relatively large abnormalities that can be seen under a microscope with special preparation of individual cells. (1) a normal pair of chromosomes; (2) an abnormality called *trisomy,* in which there is one chromosome too many; (3) part of one chromosome has been lost (or *deleted*); (4) an abnormality called a *translocation,* in which part of one chromosome has been attached to another chromosome. Most mutations cannot be seen and are studied using molecular biology techniques.

what is called a *translocation:* part of one chromosome has been rearranged and has become attached to another chromosome. What may happen here is that a regulatory region of one gene may end up on the wrong gene (the translocation may put the regulatory region of one gene next to the translated region of another). This may mean that a gene is turned on at the wrong time. If the gene is a cell cycle checkpoint gene, a cell may undergo cell division at the wrong time.

Keep these different kinds of abnormalities—trisomy, deletion, translocation, and gene silencing—in mind as you read the material that follows. When these abnormalities occur in a crucial place in the genetic material, the risk of cancer is increased. Many gene abnormalities are too subtle to be detected in a karyotype analysis and require special molecular biology techniques.

A technique called *FISH (fluorescent in situ hybridization),* al-

lows all of the chromosomes to be observed. There is a color reagent for each chromosome, so if one piece of a chromosome
is attached to another (translocation) it can be seen, assuming it
is a sufficiently large piece. Advanced technology has led to the
technique *SKY/M-FISH* (*spectral karotyping, multiplex flourescence in
situ hybridization*). SKY/M-FISH and CGH (*comparative genomic hybridization*) allow for the advanced study of cancer cytogenetics.
Computer image processing makes this possible. There are public databases through which scientists share their information. For
example, the SKY/M-FISH and CGH database can be found at
www.ncbi.nlm.nih.gov/projects/sky.

As discussed in Chapter 2, abnormal cell division can occur
either when active oncogenes (gain-of-function) are expressed or
when tumor suppressor genes (loss-of-function) are lost. An *oncogene*, recall, is a dominant gene that can cause a cancer. Having
just one oncogene can give rise to the cancer. If "C" is the cancer-
causing gene, a person with a "CC" or "Cc" gene pair would be at
risk, whereas a person with a "cc" gene pair would not. Most cancer genes that have been isolated, however, are tumor suppressor
genes; in this case, for a risk of cancer to develop, both normal
genes must be lost. In other words, the risk of cancer occurs because there is no normal gene present. If "N" is the normal gene,
a person with a "NN" or "Nn" gene pair would not be at risk, because the normal gene, "N," is present. Only a person who has a
"nn" gene pair would be at risk.

For a person who has the alleles "NN" to be at risk for a specific
cancer, *both* genes would have to be inactivated by a mutation, by
gene silencing, or by the loss of part or all of the gene—a deletion. This would require two separate events, or "hits," called the
"two-hit hypothesis." In a person with "Nn" alleles, only the "N"
gene would have to be damaged. Thus, people who are heterozygous ("Nn") are more likely to develop the cancer in their lifetime
than people who are homozygous ("NN"). Cells that retain their
heterozygosity (that continue to have a normal "N" and a "n" gene)
will not become cancerous, while a cancer cell can occur from
the "loss of heterozygosity." Because tumor suppressor genes are

usually part of normal development, it is highly unlikely that a fetus that is homozygous ("nn") would ever develop.

Gel Electrophoresis

Another method of studying genes in the laboratory uses molecular biology techniques to cut the DNA in a cell into pieces using special enzymes. The DNA is separated on a gel using a process called *gel electrophoresis*. The pieces of DNA are placed in a well on one end of the gel, and an electric current is introduced into the gel. As the pieces of DNA migrate down the gel under the pull of the electric current, the smaller pieces migrate farther than the larger pieces. The arrow in figure A.3 indicates the direction of migration.

The specific piece of DNA of interest is found by using a radioactive or fluorescent probe that will bind only to that DNA sequence (this process is called *hybridization*). The dark horizontal band in the figure indicates that the probe has bound to a specific piece of DNA on the gel.

The genes from each parent may be normal but run out differently on the gel because they may be a slightly different size. As you will recall, only part of a gene is translated into protein; there are silent areas that are not translated. Sequences of material (called *bases*) within the DNA may affect the size of the gene but not its function. Some of these sequences are called *tandem repeat sequences*. For example, within a silent, nontranscribed region, one gene may have 100 tandem repeats, whereas another may have only 50. This does not affect the genes' function, but the one with 100 is heavier and will not move as far down the gel.

Scenario 1. Detecting an abnormal gene. In this example, Offspring 1 has two normal bands, one from each parent; Offspring 2 has one normal band and one abnormal band that has a piece of DNA missing; and Offspring 3 has one band entirely missing. Offspring 1 demonstrates two bands, which indicates that the size of the gene from each parent is different (and in this case the size difference is due to the fact that each gene contains a different number of tandem repeats). [*Note:* In many situations, the band

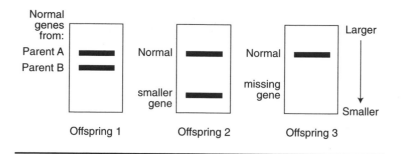

Fig. A.3. Detection of an abnormal gene using gel electrophoresis

The DNA is processed by enzymes that cut the DNA at specific spots, producing fragments of DNA of different size. The DNA is then run out on a gel that separates the fragments by size. Using a probe, a specific gene can be located. Offspring 1 demonstrates two bands because the gene from one parent is larger than the gene from the other parent. In Offspring 1, this difference in size is due to normal variation in genes called a polymorphism. In Offspring 2, because a piece of DNA is lost from one of the genes, the lower gene now migrates farther down the gel. In Offspring 3, one of the genes is missing.

from each parent is the same, so only one band will appear in the offspring (the parents' bands overlap).] In Offspring 2, note the change in the lower gene which causes it to migrate farther down the gel. In this case, a piece of the DNA has been *deleted,* so that the DNA is smaller and it migrates farther. In Offspring 3, one of the two bands has been lost: one gene is missing completely.

When the normal cells in the body have two different bands for the same gene, the pattern is heterozygous, as opposed to homozygous, when they have the same band. Scientists often compare the electrophoresis pattern from the normal cells with that of the tumor. If one of the bands is lost, it usually means that the lost band had the normal tumor suppressor gene and that the remaining band does not have a normal gene. This phenomenon is called "loss of heterozygosity," abbreviated LOH. Such an observation may not only explain why the cell became cancerous but may also help scientists discover a tumor suppressor gene.

Scenario 2. Detecting a cancer-causing gene within a family. In fig-

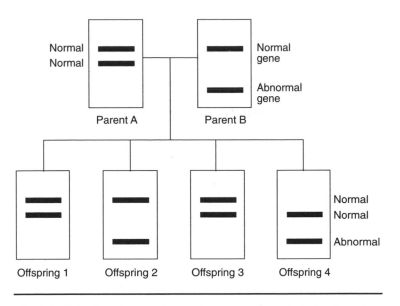

Fig. A.4. *Detection of a cancer-causing gene using gel electrophoresis*

Parent A has two different alleles of a certain gene, and both genes are normal. The gene from Parent B labeled "abnormal" has a small piece missing. Note that Parent B has passed the abnormal gene to Offspring 2 and Offspring 4.

ure A.4, Parent A has two different alleles of a certain gene, both of which are normal. They differ only in size because they contain a different number of tandem repeats. Parent B has two alleles. The top one is identical to the top one of Parent A; however, the sequence of Parent B's genes has been analyzed, and the bottom gene is known to be an abnormal gene because a small piece is missing.

As I described in Chapter 2, each child receives one gene (allele) from each parent's gene pair. Thus, among these parents' four children, Offspring 2 and Offspring 4 got the abnormal allele from Parent B and are at increased risk for cancer, whereas Offspring 1 and Offspring 3 are not at increased risk. *Note:* Offspring 2 and 4 still have one normal allele, so they do not inherit cancer, just an increased risk.

DNA Sequencing

Many abnormalities in a gene are so subtle that they don't show up in either karyotype analysis or gel electrophoresis. To study the defect, one must establish the sequence of the bases that make up the gene. DNA is made up of four bases: adenine, quanine, cytosine, and thymidine (AGCT). These bases make up the genetic code. It is now possible to sequence all of the bases within a gene. Commercial laboratories have been established which analyze genes to determine whether a person is at risk for cancer.

Genes can be extremely large, ranging up to many thousands of base pairs. To determine whether an abnormality is present in a gene, it may be necessary to sequence either the entire gene or only certain segments called "hot spots," which are prone to mutation. Although certain mutations may be harmless, others can be extremely harmful. The process of gene sequencing may identify abnormalities, some of which are crucially important to gene function and others which are not. Many genes appear to behave perfectly normally despite having slight abnormalities. These minor differences, often in a single base, are called *polymorphisms*. There is now a major effort underway to categorize polymorphisms.

Studying the Properties of Cancer Cells

All cells have a variety of proteins on their surface. Some of these cells are *lineage specific*, meaning that all cells of that type in the body have an identical protein. For example, lymph cells have different surface proteins than cells lining the stomach. In other cases, a surface protein may just be present on the cancer cells. This occurrence, though rare, would provide an excellent target for therapy.

Immunohistochemistry

Using molecules called *monoclonal antibodies*, which have a fluorescent tag, a pathologist can study a tissue section using a panel of antibodies that can help determine the tissue type of the cancer—that is, can help identify lineage-specific proteins. This is very helpful for identifying cancers that are poorly differentiated (which makes it difficult to determine the cell of origin under the microscope). The procedure of using monoclonal antibodies for diagnosis, illustrated in figure A.5, is called *immunohistochemistry*.

Polymerase Chain Reaction

Specific genes within a cancer cell can also be studied. In the technique called *polymerase chain reaction* (or *PCR*), a very, very small amount of DNA can be amplified so that there is enough to analyze. At times, it may be useful to study mRNA. Remember that a gene that is "on" in a cell makes mRNA, which then directs the cell to make the protein. Therefore, when analyzing mRNA, only the genes that are active are analyzed. Because mRNA is not very stable and is hard to work with, a technique called *reverse transcriptase–PCR* (or *RT-PCR*) is used; in this technique, mRNA is converted to DNA by an enzyme, and the DNA is then amplified and studied (see figure A.5).

In prostate cancer, for example, the technique is used as follows: Only prostate cells make a protein called *PSA*, or *prostate specific antigen*. If there are prostate cancer cells in the bone marrow because of metastases, these can be detected using RT-PCR to detect PSA. Since no normal bone marrow cells make PSA, finding PSA in the marrow indicates that a tumor in the prostate has metastasized to the bone. Finding that the cancer has already spread to bone would be important in determining treatment.

Genomics, Proteomics, and Other "Omics"

Perhaps one of the biggest revolutions in cancer research has been the development of techniques that allow scientists to study many thousands of genes and proteins at the same time. The techniques utilize basic molecular biology and protein chemistry techniques, robotics, and computer analysis.

Figure A.6 illustrates the use of DNA *microarrays* based on the property of DNA that a strand of DNA will find its appropriate other strand (pairing) due to the chemical bonds between strands.

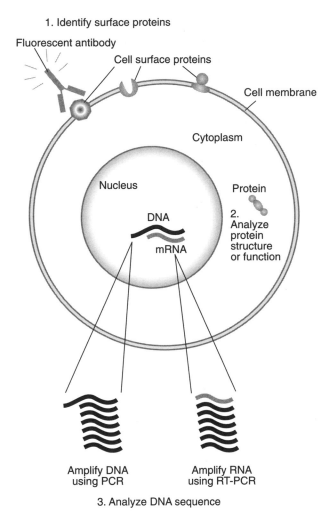

1. Identify surface proteins

Fluorescent antibody

Cell surface proteins

Cell membrane

Cytoplasm

Nucleus

Protein

DNA

2. Analyze protein structure or function

mRNA

Amplify DNA using PCR

Amplify RNA using RT-PCR

3. Analyze DNA sequence

This will occur even if there is a mixture containing many pieces of DNA. A microarray is produced by robotics. There are small pieces of DNA or parts of genes on exact locations or spots on the array. A single microarray can hold thousands of these pieces, making it possible to study thousands of genes at the same time. By comparing the microarray samples from a normal cell and a cancer cell, the processes that are involved in the cancer cell abnormality can be elucidated.

The patient's cancer cells are processed as in figure A.5 so that the mRNA is amplified and reverse transcribed into DNA. These DNA fragments are tagged with a red color reagent so that they are identified as being from the cancer cell. Another sample of a normal cell is treated the same way. This may be from the patient or from a mixed sample of many people without cancer. These are labeled green. The red and green labeled pieces of DNA are mixed and hybridized onto the microarray. If the gene from the cancer cell is there in excess of the normal cell, then a spot will be red. If the amount of gene expression in the cancer cell is less than the normal cell, the spot will appear green. If they are there in equal amounts, it will appear yellow (the equal mixture of red

---

Fig. A.5. Techniques for studying immunologic and molecular properties of cells (opposite)

Monoclonal antibodies can be used to indicate what proteins are on the surface of a cell. This can be used to distinguish one type of cell from another. For some cancers, it is not easy to be certain of the cell of origin by looking under the microscope. The use of monoclonal antibodies with an attached fluorescent tag is helpful to the pathologist in determining the cell type, a procedure called immunohistochemistry. It is possible to study very small amounts of DNA or mRNA by using an amplification process. This is called polymerase chain reaction (PCR) or, for mRNA, RT-PCR (reverse transcriptase–PCR). These techniques are used to study the specific genes in a cancer cell. They are also used for detecting a very small amount of cells in the bone marrow to check for metastases (say, from prostate cancer) or to see if some leukemia cells remain in a marrow that looks normal under the microscope.

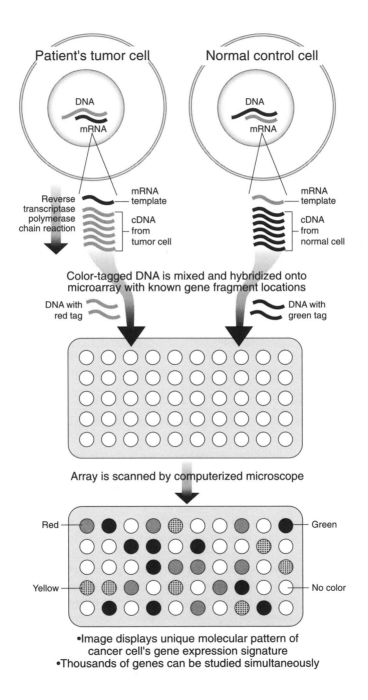

Patient's tumor cell

Normal control cell

DNA

mRNA

DNA

mRNA

Reverse transcriptase polymerase chain reaction

mRNA template

cDNA from tumor cell

mRNA template

cDNA from normal cell

Color-tagged DNA is mixed and hybridized onto microarray with known gene fragment locations

DNA with red tag

DNA with green tag

Array is scanned by computerized microscope

Red

Green

Yellow

No color

•Image displays unique molecular pattern of cancer cell's gene expression signature
•Thousands of genes can be studied simultaneously

and green produces yellow). If neither is there, the spot will be blank. This technique can detect a 1.5-fold or more difference in gene expression. Of course, meticulous technique is needed, and the presence of the abnormal gene in the cancer cell should be confirmed by other molecular biology techniques.

Scientists have discovered certain patterns of gene expression in various diseases that can predict if a cancer will be more or less

---

Fig. A.6. Microarrays for studying genes

When a gene is turned on, or expressed, the DNA makes mRNA. Using various techniques with the reverse transcriptase polymerase chain reaction shown in the figure, the mRNA is used as the template to create a larger amount of cDNA, which is more stable. The DNA can be marked with a colored molecule; in this example, the amplified DNA from the cancer cell is marked red and that of the normal cell is marked green.

Using robotics, an array is spotted at each spot with a known sequence of DNA. This can be a small piece of DNA from a gene or a synthesized piece of DNA, called an *oligonucleotide*. Based on the strength of chemical bonds between one strand of DNA and its appropriate partner strand, DNA will find its appropriate mate in a process called hybridization. The mixture of colored DNAs from the cancer and normal cell are mixed and hybridized to the array. The array is then scanned with a computerized microscope and the image is processed. What is seen are thousands of spots—red, green, yellow, or blank spots. The red spots indicate that the cancer cell had more of the gene product than the normal cell; the green spot indicates the opposite, that the normal cell had more than the cancer cell; the yellow spot means that they had equal amounts of the gene product; and the blank spots show that neither cell contained the gene.

This technique produces a molecular signature of the cancer; that is, it shows what genes are on or off compared to a normal cell. It is possible to quantify the difference in amount of gene expression (for example, three-fold overexpression or five-fold underexpression). The genes are further classified according to the pathway they are in, recognizing that some genes may function in more than one metabolic pathway and that each pathway contains many gene products. The molecular signature can be used for prognosis, to predict what therapy might work, and to help select a molecular-targeted drug (see Chapter 7).

aggressive. Treatment selection will use such information. Thus, treatment is based on the "signature" or "profile" of the patient's tumor.

Other techniques are available to study proteins (*proteomics*). These techniques can detect proteins in the blood and may be useful for cancer screening and as a form of biomarker for following a patient to see if treatment is working. Other proteomic techniques can be used to tell which signaling pathways are on, which proteins are in an active conformation, and which proteins are associated with one another.

The term "omics" is often used to refer to these general types of techniques. For example, *metabolomics* measures the cellular metabolites. These techniques allow scientists to study the complex network of the cell much more rapidly than in the past.

Analyzing Cost-Effectiveness

In this appendix, some of the basic terms and concepts used in the field of cost-effectiveness are defined. For more information on this topic I recommend two excellent articles, one by Dr. Allan Detsky, the other by Dr. Thomas Smith, both of which are listed in the bibliography.

Terms Used in the Study of Cost-Effectiveness

Charges. The amount of money charged to the insurance company or the patient. Charges are different from the amount of money actually paid. Charges for a specific procedure or test can be more or less than the cost (see below).

Cost. The actual amount spent to provide care, including personnel, facilities, and equipment.

Life expectancy (effectiveness). The average number of years a person is expected to live after receiving a certain treatment.

Life year. The amount of time gained for an entire population (called a *cohort*) as the result of a specific intervention, such as screening, a preventive measure, or a medical treatment. For example, one life year could mean that among 26 patients, all of the patients gained 2 weeks, or that 1 patient gained an entire year and 25 gained nothing.

Resource utilization. Units of medical care used to provide services. These can be converted into costs.

Utility value. A patient's estimate (derived from a standard questionnaire or research instrument) of his or her quality of life after treatment. For example, a utility value of 1 means a normal year, whereas a utility value of 0.8 means that the average person would consider each year after treatment to be equal in quality to 80 percent of the quality of a normal year.

The following calculation can be made using the above data: *Quality-adjusted life year (QALY)* equals the amount of years lived times the utility value. For example, if a treatment results in 4.5 years of life (effectiveness), with a utility value of 0.8, then the number of quality-adjusted life years is 4.5 × 0.8, or 3.6 QALYs. Another treatment might have an effectiveness of 3.5 years and a utility value of 0.9. Thus, the number of quality-adjusted life years would be calculated by multiplying 3.5 by 0.9; the result would be 3.15 QALYs.

Comparing the Cost-Effectiveness of Different Treatments

The analysis of cost-effectiveness is generally used to compare different treatments rather than to make a definitive statement about a single treatment. Incremental cost-effectiveness ratio and incremental cost-utility ratio are the calculations that are most commonly performed.

Incremental cost-effectiveness ratio is the difference in cost between two treatments (A and B in this case) divided by the difference in life expectancy:

$$\frac{[\text{Cost of treatment A} - \text{Cost of treatment B}]}{[\text{Life expectancy for treatment A} - \text{Life expectancy for treatment B}]} = \text{Dollars per life year gained}$$

Incremental cost-utility ratio is the difference in cost between two treatments divided by the difference in quality-adjusted life years:

$$\frac{[\text{Cost of treatment A} - \text{Cost of treatment B}]}{[\text{QALY for treatment A} - \text{QALY for treatment B}]} = \text{Dollars per QALY gained}$$

The current reality of health care delivery and expenditures is such that these analyses are now used to determine what resources will be made available — that is, to determine health care policy. Clearly, accurate data must used in the calculation in order for a correct conclusion to be reached. This analysis is extremely difficult to apply for an individual patient, because average values for life expectancy and utility cannot be used to predict how well a specific patient will do. The government or an insurance company might use these data to determine which treatments are appropriate and how much reimbursement will be given to the health care facility or doctor.

Performance Status Scoring Systems

Table A.1. EGOC Performance Status

Grade	ECOG
0	Fully active, able to carry on all pre-disease performance without restriction
1	Restricted in physically strenuous activity but ambulatory and able to carry out work of a light or sedentary nature, e.g., light house work, office work
2	Ambulatory and capable of all self care, but unable to carry out any work activities. Up and about more than 50% of waking hours
3	Capable of only limited self care, confined to bed or chair more than 50% of waking hours
4	Completely disabled. Cannot carry on any self care. Totally confined to bed or chair
5	Dead

Source: Oken, M. M., R. H. Creech, D. C. Tormey, J. Horton, T. E. Davis, E. T. McFadden, and P. P. Carbone, "Toxicity and Response Criteria of the Eastern Cooperative Oncology Group," *American Journal of Clinical Oncology* 5 (1982): 649–55.

*Table A.2. Karnofsky Performance Status Scale Definitions Rating (%)
Criteria*

Able to carry on normal activity and to work; no special care needed	100	Normal; no complaints; no evidence of disease
	90	Able to carry on normal activity; minor signs or symptoms of disease
	80	Normal activity with effort; some signs or symptoms of disease
Unable to work; able to live at home and care for most personal needs; varying amount of assistance needed	70	Cares for self; unable to carry on normal activity or to do active work
	60	Requires occasional assistance, but is able to care for most of his personal needs
	50	Requires considerable assistance and frequent medical care
Unable to care for self; requires equivalent of institutional or hospital care; disease may be progressing rapidly	40	Disabled; requires special care and assistance
	30	Severely disabled; hospital admission is indicated although death not imminent
	20	Very sick; hospital admission necessary; active supportive treatment necessary
	10	Moribund; fatal processes progressing rapidly
	0	Death

Source: Schrag, C. C., R. L. Heinrich, and P. A. Ganz, "Karnofsky Performance Status Revisited: Reliability, Validity, and Guidelines," *Journal of Clinical Oncology* 2 (1984): 187–93.

Patient's Checklist

Your name and address:_____

_____

_____

Your primary doctor's name and specialty:_____

_____

_____

The names of other doctors involved in your care:_____

_____

_____

_____

Diagnosis

Type of tumor and tumor site:_____

_____

_____

Clinical Staging Studies

Clinical stage:_____

_____

_____

_____

Blood tests:_____

_____

_____

_____

_____

Imaging studies:_____

_____

_____

_____

_____

Pathological Staging Studies

Pathological stage:_____

_____

_____

_____

Additional biopsies:_____

_____

_____

_____

Treatment Options

Surgery

Extent of procedure and length of hospitalization:_____

_____

_____

Side effects:_____

_____

_____

Expected results:_____

_____

_____

Radiation therapy

Region of the body to be treated:_____

_____

_____

Duration of treatment:_____

_____

_____

Side effects:_____

_____

_____

Expected results:_____

_____

_____

Systemic therapy

Drugs or agents to be used or considered:_____

_____

_____

Treatment schedule:_____

_____

_____

Hospitalization required?_____

_____

_____

Side effects:_____

_____

_____

Expected results:_____

_____

_____

Combination therapy

Sequence if this option is used:_____

_____

_____

Clinical trial

Type of treatment:_____

_____

_____

Summary of Treatment Options

_____

_____

_____

_____

Final Plan

_____

_____

_____

_____

Bibliography

Important Web site references are included within the chapters. Chapter 1 includes a table titled "Other Sources of Information" that you may find helpful.

Buckman, Robert. 1997. *What You Really Need to Know about Cancer: A Comprehensive Guide for Patients and Their Families.* Baltimore: Johns Hopkins University Press.

Cassileth, Barrie R., and Christopher C. Chapman. 1996. Alternative and complementary cancer therapies. *Cancer* 77:1026–34.

Detsky, Allan S., and I. Gary Maglie. 1990. A clinician's guide to cost-effectiveness analysis. *Annals of Internal Medicine* 113:147–54.

DeVita, Vincent T., Samuel Hellman, and Steven A. Rosenberg. 2004. *Principles and Practice of Oncology,* 6th ed. Philadelphia: J. B. Lippincott.

Dolinger, Malin, Margaret Tempero, Ernest H. Rosenbaum, and Sean Mulvihill. 2002. *Everyone's Guide to Cancer Therapy: How Cancer Is Diagnosed, Treated, and Managed Day to Day,* 4th ed. Kansas City, Mo.: Andrew and McMeel.

Eisenberg, David M. 1997. Advising patients who seek alternative medical therapy. *Annals of Internal Medicine* 127:61–69.

Hanahan, Douglas, and Robert A. Weinberg. 2000. The hallmarks of cancer. *Cell* 100:50–77.

Moore, Malcolm J., Brian O'Sullivan, and Ian F. Tannock. 1988. How expert physicians would wish to be treated if they had genitourinary cancer. *Journal of Clinical Oncology* 6:1736–45.

Smith, Thomas J., Bruce E. Hillner, and Christopher E. Desch. 1993. Efficacy and cost-effectiveness of cancer treatment: Rational allocation of resources based on decision analysis. *Journal of the National Cancer Institute* 85:1460–74.

Index

About the Author

Dr. C. Norman Coleman received his medical degree from Yale University School of Medicine. He subsequently completed residencies in internal medicine at the University of California in San Francisco; medical oncology at the National Cancer Institute, National Institutes of Health in Bethesda, Maryland; and radiation oncology at Stanford University Medical School in Stanford, California. He is board certified in all three medical specialties.

After completing his medical training, he joined the faculty at Stanford, where he achieved the rank of associate professor with tenure of medicine (medical oncology) and radiology (radiation oncology). From 1985 to 1999 he served as the Alvin T. and Viola D. Fuller–American Cancer Society Professor at Harvard Medical School and chairman of the Joint Center for Radiation Therapy, which served five Harvard teaching hospitals and a regional community network throughout Massachusetts. In 1999, he returned to the National Cancer Institute in a program he created, the Radiation Oncology Sciences Program, that includes patient care, physics and biology research, and oversight of the radiation oncology/biology grant program. He also serves as special advisor to the director of NCI. He is a senior medical advisor in the Office of Public Health Emergency Preparedness, U.S. Department of Health and Human Services, working on a program to develop medical countermeasures for radiation injury and exposure.

Dr. Coleman maintains an active clinical practice that involves innovative multimodality approaches to diagnosis and treatment. He has served on a number of academic, oncology society, and government advisory boards, on the editorial board of PDQ–Physicians Data Query of NCI, and as a reviewer for a variety of oncology journals. Along with his colleagues at NCI, he is involved in novel pro-

grams to bring clinical research advances to underserved popula-
tions within the United States and internationally. Among his many
honors and named lectures, he has been awarded the Gold Medal
of the American Society of Therapeutic Radiology and Oncology
(ASTRO).